MICH

PHALLUS

THE HISTORY OF AN OBSESSION

Cover photo: Renaissance lads, the summit of male beauty and virility.

''The heart has reasons reason will never know.''
Pascal

© 2017

In Caesar's *Commentaries* he said this about autoeroticism: ''To the lonely it is company; to the forsaken it is a friend; to the aged and impotent it is a benefactor; they that be penniless are still rich, in that they have this majestic diversion. There are even times when I prefer it to sodomy.''

The pornographic film *Kansas City Trucking Co.* is all about masturbation, which Gage explains in this way: ''The whole idea of making homosexual pornography... [if] you strip it down to its absolute basics, [which is] the worship of the phallus, the worship of the penis. If you're going to make homosexual pornography, you'd better highlight the penis-- that's what it's about.''

Dr Samuel-Auguste Tissot's *Thesis on Masturbation*--''self-pollution and its polluting consequences''--ruined the adolescence of uncountable boys, including my own, from its inception in 1758 to the advent of the Internet.

When pressed by reporters to explain why the United States was involved in Vietnam, LBJ whipped out his penis and said, ''*This* is why!''
From Robert Dallek's *Flawed Giant: Lyndon Johnson and His times, 1961-1973.*

In 2009 Spain spent a whopping €14,000 on a campaign with the slogan ''Pleasure Is In Your Own Hands'', aimed at promoting masturbation in the age category 14 to 17.

''Always buy pornographic books in hardback because they're easier to hold with one hand.''
Robert Clark

''Mankind is governed by the Fates, even the private parts clothes conceal; if the stars are against you the fantastic size of your member will get you nowhere.''
Juvenal – 1st century A.D.

Marlon Brando advised boys
to always go in the direction their erect dick pointed: it *never* makes mistakes.

''You cannot blame porn. When I was young, I used to masturbate to *Gilligan's Island*.'' [*Gilligan's Island* was an American sitcom about two crewmembers and five passengers shipwrecked on a Pacific Ocean island.]

''He was thinking with his other head,'' someone said about why Clinton had sex with a White House intern, despite the fact that the second head lacked the 100 billion nerve cells of the [so-called] first head.

Sophocles wrote that having a dick was equivalent to being ''chained to a madman.''

''What's good about masturbation is that you don't have to get dressed for it.''
Truman Capote

''God gave every man a brain and a penis but only enough blood to make one work at a time.''
Actor Robin Williams

To sow your seed go naked, strip to plow and strip to reap, thus each crop will come in turn.
Hesiod *Works and Days*

Da Vinci wrote that a woman's desire was the opposite of a man's, as she wanted him large and he wanted her narrow.

Cecil Beaton said to Garbo, ''With age my privates are shrinking.'' Answered the Devine: ''If only I could say the same for mine.''

''Don't knock masturbation. It's sex with someone you love.''
Woody Allen

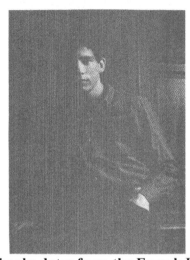

The inspiration of my books dates from the French Revolution with its Declaration of the Rights of Man in 1789, the end of homophobia in 1791, followed by the right of each man to marry the boy of his choice in 2013, the whole confirmed, in the States, by the American Supreme Court. My books include: *Cellini, Caravaggio, Cesare Borgia, Renaissance Murders, TROY, ARGO, Greek Homosexuality, Roman Homosexuality, Renaissance Homosexuality, Alcibiades the Schoolboy, RENT BOYS, Henry III, Louis XIII, Buckingham, Homoerotic Art (in full color), Sailors and Homosexuality, The Essence of Being Gay, John (Jack) Nicholson, THE SACRED BAND, Prussian Homosexuality, Gay Genius, SPARTA, Charles XII of Sweden, Mediterranean Homosexual Pleasure, CAPRI, Boarding School Homosexuality, HUSTLERS, Tasmania, American Homosexual Giants* and *Christ has his John, I have my George: The History of British Homosexuality.* I live in the South of France.

http://www.amazon.com/author/mbhone
http://www.amazon.com/Michael-Hone/e/B00J7UOHQC

CONTENTS

INTRODUCTION

BEGINNINGS
Min
Enki
Uranus
Eros
Page 9

INTRODUCTION

When I left my native Mormon Utah and the U.S.A. at age 18 I had never heard the ''f''-word pronounced orally, and the most erotic reference to the male appendage had come when I entered my junior-high-school locker room and someone said to me, looking towards my midsection, ''Your hobby's open.'' When I looked down at my levis fly the guy continued, ''So *that's* your hobby!'' The guys standing around broke out in laughter, I turned deeply red, totally unsuspecting of the great happiness my hobby had in store for me on my arrival at Cherbourg, the gateway to Europe (1).

As hard as marble, upright like a spur, a sword, a dagger, the giver of infinite pleasure and unique procreator, a source of immense comfort at boyhood, perhaps even a boy's very first true happiness, free, disinterested and supremely loyal. In dark moments, who better to turn to for solace? Stress vanishes, the body is wracked by a wondrous sensation, and the visible proof of manhood, the lakes and rivers covering the still-shuddering abdomen, glisten amidst the sweat. It is a boy's first and only true mate, one the boy will share with glee, but even after an evening of wild debauch, it'll return home with the guy that brought him. Always.

The fixation on the male member, the answer to the ''Whys'' of our obsession concerning it, and that throughout the ages, is the basis of this book.

We'll examine it through historical figures, Alcibiades for the Greeks, Priapus for the Romans, François I for France, Casanova for Venice, Byron will guide us through English Romanticism and Howard Hughes will represent America.

We'll learn how to length it, to *really* lengthen it, and how to restore the foreskin of those mutilated in infancy. We'll discover the benefits of that purist of elixirs, semen. Male nudity throughout time will be developed-- how boys displayed their assets in Greek gymnasiums and Roman baths, baths in which men generously endowed were applauded, to the Renaissance where boys were the most brazen in their public eroticism, followed by pre-Elizabethan codpieces, and today's jocks and briefs.

I'll be using the word phallus as a synonym for penis, although a phallus is often an erect penis. My preference goes to the ''c''-word c**k, but if I use it this book will be restricted to an adult public only. The same is true with the ''f''-word, that I'll replace with something milder. Autoeroticism will be used in place of masturbation because the lies concerning it, that had me sweating bullets of guilt during my adolescence, have poisoned the word forever in my mind.

I use numerals when I think a number is important--especially age milestones--because they stand out more clearly, no matter how big or small the number. Also, there will be a certain number of statistics used throughout this book, concerning penis dimensions, frequency of sexual contacts, infidelity averages, down to the distance a boy can climax through autoeroticism, from dribbling over the knuckles to well over his head. They *all* rarely concord, although, generally, they are in the same ballpark, the reason I'm giving them. That said, we can only hope that somewhere in the world a follow-up study to the Kinsey Report is underway, one that will fully include the immense, truly immense, sexual influence of Internet.

BEGINNINGS
Min
Enki
Uranus
Eros

Enki

Enki, Lord of Life, was the god of Ab, meaning water and semen in Sumerian. It was written in 3000 B.C.:

Enki, eyeing the Euphrates,
Stood lustfully like a bull,
Stroked his phallus to ejaculate,
Filling the Euphrates with flowing water.

And later:

He lifted his phallus like a wild bull,
And gave birth to the Tigris.

Still erect, he used his hardness to plough the fields between the two rivers, providing food for the race he then fathered, and sang out, ''Let my phallus now be praised!''

The fertilizing power from his water was so strong that vegetation sprang up everywhere, and girls were forbidden to bathe least they become pregnant. Enki himself drank his water, his semen, and himself became pregnant. His people watched helpless as he swelled up, fearing for his life because he had no womb. But his wife took pity on him and absorbed the child into her own body.

Min

Min was an early Egyptian god dating from the 4th millennium and was represented with an ever-erect phallus. He was honored yearly by the pharaoh who ejaculated into the Nile, thusly assuring its fertility through the annual flooding. The symbols of Min were a white bull and lettuce, which was considered an aphrodisiac because it produced a milky semen-like substance. Without the pharaoh's phallus and ejaculate the Nile would become infertile and the Egyptians doomed to death by starvation.

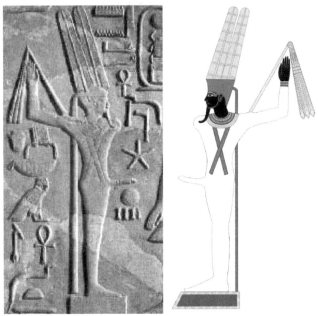

The pharaoh himself, represented here, was the source of regeneration and resurrection.

Osiris

Osiris was the god of the Afterlife, the guarantor of Resurrection. The son of the sun god Ra [or Re], brother and husband of Isis, father of Horus, Horus who was both begot and born posthumously.

Osiris was murdered by his brother Seth who took his throne. Seth dismembered the body that Isis was able to collect, after complicated searches, except for the phallus supposedly eaten by Nile fish. One version had Isis construct a new phallus from wood that she integrated to the body she then mummified, the first mummification in Egyptian history. She brought Osiris back to life, the time to become pregnant with Horus, and through Osiris's resurrection opened the way for eternal life for everyone who would subscribe to certain sacred ceremonies.

As for Seth, Horace killed him and hacked off his virile member, which Egyptians would then perpetuate in battle, the Pharaoh Merneptah taking, as trophies, the members of 6 Lybian generals and 6,359 soldiers during a war against Libyans in 1200 B.C.

Osiris eventually merged Ra with Atum to become Atum-Ra, king of the gods, father of pharaohs. Atum had created the Nile with masturbatory ejaculate, as Enki had done.

The Phoenicians called their chief god Asshur from their word Asher meaning phallus, the Upright, the Powerful, the Opener, he who ruptures the hymen in the first coition with a virgin.

Semen is life's purest elixir, from which, when fired by desire, all life springs forth. Enki filled the Tigris and Euphrates. The sperm of Min created the Nile. And Shiva's seed conceived the Ganges.

Uranus

Uranus was the sky, who covered the Earth, Gaia, each night, impregnating her with children that were forced to remain within the mother by the oppressive weight of Uranus's body. Suffering terrible pain, Gaia produced a sickle and begged her sons to use it to free her from Uranus. Her youngest, most ambitious boy, Cronus, agreed to undertake the task if he could become the first of the gods. Gaia agreed and Cronus, sickle in hand, grasped this father Uranus's testicles and phallus and severed all with one huge stroke, the blood released forming the gods, and from the phallus sprange Aphrodite. Cronus was later imprisoned in Tartarus by his son Zeus.

Eros

There is another version of Aphrodite's origin, that I've lifted from my book *TROY*:

A handsome redheaded lad carrying a quiver on his back and a gold bow in his hand flew slowly towards them. Eros was of an age as yet untroubled by the havoc his arrows wrought, but he was amenable, as the poet said, to girls who would persuade him to play night games with them, laughing knowingly when he did as they asked.

"You look dog tired, adorable Eros," said Eos.

"I had a full night's work," smirked the god of Passion. "The weekends are really becoming insupportable. Orgies and onanism, secret assignations and happenstance encounters, bacchanals and banquets; not to speak of ordinary necking and necrophilia, seduction and sadism."

"I admire your handiwork, lovable Eros," said Helios. "And you're always so successful!"

"What god wouldn't be a success packing this quiver of love darts around? Is there a boy who does not awaken to my sting before his voice becomes that of a man? To my sting what maiden does not succumb to the lovesick eyes of her young pursuer? I am the eternal beginning, the everlasting renaissance, the glorious spring."

"Next you'll tell us that you're the most important of the gods," observed Eos.

"As the first-born I have all the rights," scorned Eros, blood rushing to his ruddy cheeks. "In a family is not the first-born the most anticipated of children? Is he not the most ardent of a maiden's yearning and the great proof of her mate's virility? And when the first-born grows to manhood, is it not he, by law, who is responsible for his brothers and sisters and yea, must he not answer for the conduct of his mother and support her and her children and the household and servants and slaves when his father goes to war? Or if his father falls in battle, must he not take in charge his mother's and brothers' suitors and his sisters' dowries? Should he then not be the most respected and cuddled, the most honored and revered? Yes, say I."

"And I too, beautiful Eros," said Helios.

"As do I," seconded Eos. "We respect our little Eros, my brother and I. But we are in the minority. The other gods adore but do not adorn you. They think you--I hope you will not find this offensive and thereby wish to take revenge upon me--irresponsible, if not to say perverse."

"Oh! The ungrateful lot!" smoldered Eros.

"Perhaps, dearest Eros. No! Surely, I mean," said Helios, redressing his awkwardness. "They surely are as you have said, ungrateful. And worse. Much worse. But wasn't it you and those love-tipped arrows of yours that brought forth from the union of Mother Earth and Tartarus the hideous god Typhon? Did you not push Thyestes to ravish Pelopia, his own daughter? Did not Apollo, mad with lust, take as lover Hyacinth--the first god to be united in ungodly lust with not only a mere mortal, but a boy?"

"As if you, Helios, did not crave for the sweet company of..."

"No, no, don't interrupt me, you wicked child!" Helios would have blushed were his coloring not already a brilliant gold. "What god is not driven to perversion by your silly whims and your ... your..." he sputtered, losing the thread of his thoughts. He ran his amber fingers through the bronze curls of his beard. "Where was I..."

" Hyacinth?" suggest Eos.

"Ah, yes. Thanks Sister. Hyacinth. And these are just some of the innumerable stories about your improprieties. Pushed by Passion, men have killed, shacked up with beasts, committed incest and have been driven to suicide. No horror is above your imagination, no abomination is beyond your capability, no sanctity is safe from your need to defile. In short, you're a scoundrel, darling Eros, a knave and a rascal, dearest, beautiful Eros."

"You wish me to be offended brother sun, but I'm thick-skinned and even if I did harbor some slight resentment against you, I would need but wait until you beg me for one of my favors without which you would spend your nights alone and loveless. I know that the gods--like the mortals--are ungrateful and never satisfied. All of you blame your woes on Eros, the first of the gods, for without me there would have been no inclination to produce others."

"How were you born, marvelous Eros?" inquired Eos. "It's been so long since I left school that I've totally forgotten the History of the Beginning of Time."

"My parents," began Eros, eager to take the stage, "were Mother Desire and Father Deviation, two old gods dethroned by the new ones. All I remember is awaking in the middle of a pile of egg shells where the ocean laps against the shore." In his mind's eye he saw the long crescent beach with its tepid sands and lucent waters. His birth had been a moment of such divine ecstasy that he carried its sweet imprint throughout the whole of his eventful, carefree life.

"And at birth you found yourself completely on your own?" asked Helios.

"Yes, and as a god I was full-grown when only nine days old. I was very curious and since I was alone, I had only myself to play with. One day, therefore, as I was taking in the warmth of a brilliant afternoon and pursuing solitary amusement in the hollow of some rocks a few feet above the sea, I gave myself up to the most voluptuous of feelings, and low and behold from the place where my seed splattered upon the crystal waters rose up the most beautiful of women, naked and enthroned in a scallop shell. She rode on the foam of little wavelets that placed her ever so gently upon the sand. We immediately became great friends and discovered that we had a good deal in common: I, Eros, god of Passion and she, Aphrodite-- for such was her name--the goddess of Love. And as you know, we were made it hit-it-off and hit-it-off we did and always have."

Aphrodite's attraction was to both men and boys, from the roughest, the god of War Ares, to sweet Hermes, as we see in this scene from *TROY*. Eros, to get revenge because his creation, Aphrodite, voted against his entry into the Olympic Godhead, has Helios, the sun, inform Aphrodite's husband, the misshapen Hephaestus, that his wife was in the throes of love with one of her many paramours:

Everyone who was anyone on Olympus was there: The Twelve Ruling Gods with notably Zeus from Olympus, Hades from Tartarus and Poseidon from Ocean; the Three Fates, the Cyclopes, the Dactyls; the heroes: Theseus, Perseus and Heracles; Lapiths and Centaurs and Minotaurs; the Winds, the Furies, the Planets; Night, Day and Mother Earth; as well as uncountable other lesser gods, monsters, servants and sycophants.

Those with a modicum of modesty and virtue remained outside; the others were within, fighting for a view. As was only proper, the greater gods like Zeus and his favorite son Hermes, Apollo, Poseidon and of course Hephaestus himself had ringside seats. Eros was still there and had been joined by Dionysus.

What they saw on the massive couch was an outraged Aphrodite and a rather silly-looking Ares, both firmly ensnared in a finely-forged bronze net that Hephaestus had fashioned. Like Aphrodite, Hephaestus was beside himself with anger: "You Thracian slut, you Egyptian harlot, you Trojan whore; this is the last time you're going to make a fool of me," he howled in humiliation.

"Buckle your warty mouth, you little runt," cried out Aphrodite, crimson with mortification. "No one's making a fool of you but you yourself."

"We're divorcing and that goat that's humping you is going to repay every drachma of dowry," yelled Hephaestus, and then broke down in tears.

Poseidon, who had instantly fallen in love with Aphrodite upon seeing her naked, came to comfort him.

"It's a god's fate to be cuckolded," whispered Poseidon.

"The sniveling lecher!" sobbed Hephaestus.

"And we have to be philosophical about it," continued Poseidon. "It's an accident that has befallen even the best of us. The thing to do now is to repair the damage. As your good friend I promise to make Ares pay you back the equivalent of your marriage gifts," declared beguiling Poseidon.

"And if he doesn't?" sniffed Hephaestus.

"If he doesn't, why, for the love of you I'll take his place under the net and reimburse you myself."

"Good enough," said Hephaestus, blowing his nose.

"What do you think of Aphrodite?" whispered Apollo to Hermes. "Wouldn't you like to be in Ares's place now?"

"I'll say I would," answered the very excited Hermes. "I'll marry Aphrodite myself if Hephaestus really divorces her, and if she would want me."

Aphrodite was listening, and a long time afterwards, in another place, she would bestow her ample favors on young Hermes, from which union would be born, by and by, Hermaphrodite.

"Oh, Eros," sighed Dionysus, up from Naxos for the occasion, "have you ever seen anything more beautiful? I am in love--now and forever!"

Aphrodite who, as the Olympians say, doesn't have her ears in her pockets, heard this too. Later on Priapus, an obscenely ugly child with enormous genitals, was born to them.

Another woman for whom the phallus was an obsession was Helen of Troy, from *TROY*:

The evening before Helen had received the visit of Eros in the form of a young lover. Lying on her side, encircled in the warm hollow of his arms, her back against his chest, his knees tucked into hers, they had passed the night in love's embrace. He was a Trojan youth, Eros pretended, the son of a king, although his abode was a mud hut and his stepfather a herdsman. He had searched and finally found Helen, and before slipping out from the caressing folds of her bed he promised that they would be together again that night in the privacy of dreams.

"Then there's Aegisthus," Clytaemnestra was saying. "A little young, perhaps. He probably detests me, seeing that it was Agamemnon who deprived him of his throne." Her own hatred for her husband Agamemnon had long since sapped Clytaemnestra's vitality, turning her into a bitter harridan. She looked up. "You don't seem to be giving your marriage much thought."

"Why should I concern myself with the choice of a suitor?" murmured Helen, separating two lashes stuck with mascara. "It's not for me to decide."

Helen's real father was Zeus, and it was his immortal blood and Helen's awareness of it that placed her irredeemably beyond the interests of the time in which she lived. In a totally uncaring and vapid cosmos, she awaited the cataclysm that would give to her existence meaning. Helen's entire being was a mask, the Fates' own tool; she was an emissary from the gods set on dominating Man.

"Some would think you lucky," said Clytaemnestra.

"Lucky?" pouted petal-soft Helen. She picked up a silver chalice of Spartan mountain wine and took a small sip.

"Perhaps I would," remembered Clytaemnestra.

"You...?" muttered Helen, back to her mirror.

"After all, it was Agamemnon who killed my first husband..."

Yes, thought Helen, and impaled your newborn baby on his sword, as a lion kills the cubs of the lioness he lusts for. Their world was barbaric; better to bend to one's lot like wind-blown grass. To the East lay civilization, she knew, in cities such as Troy. There, no man would ever gain a hold on Helen as Agamemnon had Clytaemnestra.

There was a knock at the door. A girl of fifteen entered.

"Penelope," smiled Helen.

"Have the altars been built for the sacrifices?" asked Clytaemnestra.

"They're burning an ox in honor of Zeus and one for Hera," said Penelope. She placed herself behind Helen and began braiding the blond strands of her hair into one long golden rope.

Penelope was Helen and Clytaemnestra's adopted sister, but she was close to neither. Clytaemnestra was far too self-pitying to be able to care for the young girl, and Helen too remote. It was common knowledge that the sisters' mother, Leda, had hatched both Helen and Clytaemnestra from the same egg, one half fertilized by Tyndareus and mortal, the other half fecundated by Zeus who had taken the form of a swan, slipping its outstretched neck between Leda's open thighs as she bathed at a lake's edge. Helen was the product of this immortal half. It was the blood of Zeus that gave Helen her eternal beauty and an aloofness for things terrestrial. She shared but one destiny with mortal women--the destiny of all mortal women: that of inspiring love.

"They're the most important," said Clytaemnestra. "Don't forget Athena or Arthemis, or Apollo and ... let's see, who else? Oh yes, Eros: We can't have the wedding night go badly."

The conversation plodded on, like the wearisome ebb and flow of the sea, the three unfortunates oblivious to having overlooked Aphrodite in the sacrifices. The price they were to pay would be a thousand fold what which the goddess had extracted from Eos, forever unable to find satisfaction in the embrace of young lovers.

Helen listened to neither of them. That night she would find herself in the arms of one of the strangers in the outer room, but it was with the Trojan youth that would enter her with his Trojan massiveness.

In the dining room Calchas saw Tyndareus rise to make known his choice for son-in-law.

"You know how difficult it is today for a husband and wife with thieves, bands of murderers and wars threatening the family hearth," began the old king. "That's why I want to protect this marriage by asking each of you to take an oath supporting Helen and my pick of bridegroom from any danger wherever it may come."

In this way did Tyndareus reveal Odysseus' plan for avoiding bloodshed, and it was his reward for this plan that would later win Odysseus the fair Penelope.

"If you are all of a mind to do this," continued Tyndareus, "stand up!" The suitors, disgruntled, got to their feet. "And now promise in the name of the gods and the River Styx to protect Helen and her future bridegroom."

The oath was solemnly taken by each man. Only then did Tyndareus announce Menelaus as his choice of son-in-law.

And in her boudoir, Helen, unmoved by the haggling outside, dipped an elegant finger in the chalice of purple wine before her, and on the lacquered top of her dressing table wrote the name of her handsome lover in dreams--Paris.

We end with Aphrodite, this time at the side of the most beautiful Trojan to have lived, Paris, called upon to decide which of the three goddesses gets the Golden Apple, the awarding of which will soon ignite the Trojan War, from *TROY*:

On Earth Apollo, the youth who had intercepted Paris on his way to Troy with a sacrificial bull, introduced him to the three goddesses.

Hera had descended wearing a scarlet robe for the occasion, as well as a jeweled diadem. She carried the symbol of her godly rank, the sacred scepter, in her right hand. She put on her most dazzling smile.

Athena wore a full suit of golden armor carved by that master of all smithies, Hephaestus, and a tunic of warm Thracian wool. She, too, was grinning from ear to ear.

Aphrodite had chosen her simplest dress for the event, a silk veil made on the island of Cos from the finest imported cocoons. It fell from her throat to her ankles and no cobweb could rival its fineness. It was attached to Aphrodite at the waist by a magic girdle that made its wearer instantly loved by anyone laying eyes on it.

Athena noticed Aphrodite's dishonest advantage. "Apollo, tell her to take off her girdle; it's not fair."

The demand did not go unnoticed by Paris. The girdle was the symbol of a girl's virginity. To take it off meant she was going to offer herself. The thought turned the young man's skin noticeably red and caused his chiton to rise significantly, an embarrassment instantly noted by Aphrodite and, especially, Apollo.

"Father said there was to be no arguing," stressed Apollo, clearing his suddenly dry throat before reminding them of Zeus's oath to turn them into burnt crust if they weren't ladylike. "Paris is here to do the judging. It's for him to decide how he wants to get on with it."

"Perhaps it would be an unfair edge," said Paris, "your keeping on the belt and all. Would you mind removing it please." And then in a whisper he asked Apollo, "Do you think I could get them to disrobe? After all, how can I judge them if..."

Apollo interrupted Paris with a knowing smile and a wink. "You're the boss, Paris; they're obliged to go along with anything you say. Father's given strict orders."

"But if I offended one of them," said the boy, his back to the ladies while he adjusted the protuberance so it was held firm under the belt of the tunic, "she could strike me down in no time flat."

"Father's told them to behave themselves," said the god, obliged to do the same, his eyes glued to Paris. "But if you want to make sure, have them take an oath on the River Styx to abide by your decisions and in no way try to harm you."

Paris thought much of the advice and followed it to the letter. After the goddesses had all sworn by the Styx, Paris had them disrobe and come to him one at a time. The others hung back out of earshot to avoid arguments.

Hera was the first.

"You look like such a nice young man, Paris. Isn't it funny we haven't seen you around before? Now, I want you to think of me as if we've been friends for years. Forget that I'm the goddess Hera, queen of the Heavens and wife to Almighty Zeus, wielder of supreme power. Just look me over as you would an old friend, or a member of the family, your mother for instance. Yes, just consider me as plain old Mom. Is your mother as beautiful as I am, Paris?"

"I can't rightly tell you, ma'am. I've never seen her naked." The notion and Hera herself immediately deflated the boy's ardor.

"Well that's modern education for you. In my time clothes hadn't even been invented."

"Yes, ma'am."

"You know, Paris, I would like to do a little something for you, as one friend to another, as--for example--a mother for her son. How would you like to become emperor of all Asia and the richest human alive?"

"I'm really not that way inclined, ma'am."

"What would you like?"

"I can't rightly say."

"You've never thought about it, have you, Son?"

"No, ma'am. Not much."

"Well, you remember that Mom thinks the world of you, and in return you could make her very happy by awarding her the apple. Will you, boy?"

"I'll have to see the others first, ma'am. But you can be sure my decision will be fair and square."

Hera stepped confidently away, and up came Athena, completely uncovered except for her golden helmet, without which she lost much of her glamour.

"Would you mind turning around, Athena, so as I can get you all in," asked emboldened Paris. Athena complied resolutely with all the grace and appeal of a foot soldier.

"Please get an eyeful, Paris, and while you're taking in my charms one by one let me promise you that if you present me with the apple, I'll make you victorious in all battles and the wisest man on Earth."

"Fighting and book-learning don't interest me an awful lot, goddess, but I promise to judge you as honestly as the other two. Just please don't try to bribe me because it won't work."

Paris dismissed Athena who went striding off. She was followed by Aphrodite.

The goddess of Love had removed her girdle, but kept on her veil-like dress. Its transparency indecently revealed the flawless beauty of her perfect form. A lusty little breeze lifted the gossamer covering to divulge the youthful voluptuousness of the delicate mound between her legs; then the lecherous wind pressed the filmy veil against her body, outlining her shiny, gold-tipped breasts.

Aphrodite came very close to Paris.

"My goodness, but aren't you the handsomest," she cooed. "I just can't figure out what a boy like you is doing in a hole like this. Where do you go for excitement? What you need is the goings-on of the city, fine clothes and a woman as beautiful as you are handsome. And do you know, Paris, I've got the name of the perfect woman right here on the tip of my tongue. She's Helen of Sparta. She's as beautiful as any living mortal and nearly as beautiful as myself. I'll send you to Sparta with Eros. He'll make Helen fall head over heels for you--which in your case won't be hard. Her husband, Menelaus, is going away on a trip soon and you'll have the whole palace to yourselves."

"She's *married*!" exclaimed Paris.

"You *are* a country bumpkin, aren't you," laughed Aphrodite. "What difference does *that* make? Just because Menelaus saw her *first* doesn't mean you don't have as much right to her love as he did. But," added Aphrodite, "before sailing to Sparta you'll have to go to Troy and have Priam recognize you as his son. It's only as a prince that Menelaus will invite you into his palace. Now," she continued "about Helen. Come closer, Paris, let me describe her in detail."

Close enough to brush against his renewed manhood, Aphrodite whispered animatedly into Paris's ear while Paris blushed sheepishly at her narration. Midway through her description she gently withdrew the apple from his hands and slipped it to her faithful servant Eros for safekeeping. She then went into the particulars with Paris about how to execute her scheme.

Athena and Hera, outraged by what was going on, withdrew arm in arm to plan their revenge.

And Chaos slowly descended over Heaven and Earth, enveloping all in the black folds of her despicable robe.

Greeks and Romans didn't practice cunnilingus, and fellatio was not favored. Both preferred the gradual buildup of vaginal, anal and intercrural sex. As wall murals and mosaics prove, the Greeks and Romans had multiple sexual positions, while from Medieval times to Elizabethan, face-to-face sex was the rule, the missionary position considered the best for the flow of semen when children were desired, and remains the hands-down preference today because it allows deep kissing, the ultimate erogenous zone, and allows the boy to see the pleasure in the face of the woman submitting to his masculine domination, his body shiny from the exertion. For homosexuals it's the same, the penetrator always the more virile of the two, even when bottoms like Joey Stefano and Donovan Casey could send a guy to seventh heaven (4). Greek whores charged more when they sat on the man, the least when he took her standing in some alley, more if she was taken doggy.

Greeks today ejaculate often and fast, in 4 minutes, and a study in 2005 said the average time to reach orgasm--throughout the world--was 5.4

minutes, while homosexuals spend infinitely longer in foreplay and varied techniques, but then homosexuals often change partners, very often in fact, which is *immensely* more stimulating than driving into the same person night after night. Homosexual couples will not hesitate to invite others to share in their lovemaking, nor will they hesitate to take part in orgies together, or pool parties, or a night at the sauna [if they don't, they'll eventually separate]. It's the only way to keep the couple together, because the curiosity to find out what lies beyond new boys' unexplored jeans and briefs will always win out over fidelity. [The word orgy [ὄργια], in Greek times, referred to ecstatic religious rites that differed from public religion and private household religion in that they were secrete and open only to initiates. Taking place at night, the Romans suspected them of being sexual in nature, but in reality they were mostly ecstatic attempts to unite with the divine.]

In the sixteenth and seventeenth centuries maidens referred to their boyfriends as ''my prick,'' while at the end of the seventeenth century such words began to be replaced--apricocks, haycocks and weathercocks became apricots, haystacks and weather vanes, while in America water cocks became faucets and cocks, roosters. Men exchanged rods for yards, ''an optimistic measurement of length,'' writes Tom Hickman in his wonderful *GOD'S DOODLE*: *The Life and Times of the Penis*, 2012. Our word avocado comes from the Aztec word for scrotum.

Men have sought ways to get hard and stay that way since the dawn of time. Egyptians applied a poultice on the member, made of acacia leaves, honey and *Paliurus spina-Christi*, that we call Christ-thorn today, a prickly plant. The Assyrians ate a concoction of dried lizards and crushed beetles, while later Assyrian preferences went to a woman who rubbed the deflated member with oil and iron powder, while calling it a horse that she needed to make love to her, the massaging and the flattery apparently working miracles.

Testicles, taken in one form or another, were always popular, the Greek physician Nicander prescribing those of hippopotami, while in Rome orgies were fueled by aphrodisiacs consisting of goat and wolf testes.

Da Vinci had been one of the first [perhaps even *the* first] to conclude that erections were caused by blood flow, while doctors even into the 1800s attributed erections to ''erector muscles'' that they attempted to stimulate through electric shocks. The patient was willing to go along in hopes of improvement, but also because doctors universally believed that the cause of impotence was self-abuse, and so the patient accepted the shock punishment as merited.

During da Vinci's life it was also believed that erections were cause by air, a pneumatic force, but was dismissed by da Vinci as impossible because of the pressure of air necessary to produce such turgidity [from Dr. Marc Bonnard and Dr. Michel Schouman's book *Histoire du Pénis*, 1999].

Worse was still to come, in the form of testicle transplants [the first transplants of any human organ was a testicle sewn into the scrotum]. When human donors were unavailable, animal testes were used, the patient usually ignorant of the fact. As the microsurgery necessary to connect the nerves, tubes and blood vessels was none-existent, the improvement noticed by the patient was entirely psychological, aided by the fact that only one testicle was replaced, although a certain John R. Brinkley got rich by publicizing the benefits of a goat testicle, goats considered, since Greek and Roman times, the ideal source of virility.

John Romulus Brinkley is of great interest. He was born in 1885 to a mountain man who served as medic in the Civil War and later practiced medicine without a diploma. The mountain man's first marriage was annulled because he was underage, he outlived his wives during the four marriages that followed, and had John out of wedlock with one of his many mistresses. John married at age 22 and he and his wife, pretending to be doctors, mounted a medicine show during which he hawked virility tonics. He entered an unaccredited medical college where he learned about glands and glandular extracts. He dropped out of school, bought a diploma and opened a shop were he sold virility injections, colored water at $25 a shot [$600 today]. He left his wife and bigamously married another. [They had a son who later committed suicide.]

Brinkley opened a clinic and wrote that one of his patients complained of lacking virility in lovemaking. When Brinkley jokingly told him he needed a goat's testicle, the man begged him to implant one [the man's son later said that Brinkley had paid the man to undergo the operation, and then paid to tell one and all that it was a resounding success].

The result was an explosion of clients and Brinkley's personal wealth, as he charged $1,750 [$9,000 today] for simply posing goat gonads in scrotal sacs, where they were absorbed as foreign matter. Infections and death regularly occurred, and Brinkley faced dozens of suits.

As his fame grew, the renowned owner of the *Los Angeles Times*, Otis Chandler, summoned Brinkley to perform the operation on one of his editors, promising him fame if he succeeded, damnation if he didn't. Chandler's power was such that he got Brinkley a special permit to proceed, even though he wasn't recognized as a licensed doctor. When the operation was deemed a success, Hollywood cliental followed, including film stars.

He built his own radio station chiefly to publicize himself, and in the town where he practiced, Milford, Kansas, he introduced a sewage system, installed electricity, built a new post office, sponsored the hometown baseball team, the Brinkley Goats, offered homes to the poor, and then ran for Governor of Kansas [but lost].

Lawsuits and poor health got the best of him in 1942, when he died at age 57, penniless.

This nonsense existed too in psychoanalysts who assured patients that their problem was exclusively psychological, without ever examining them as a urologist would have done. The snag was that, at the time, the urologists might themselves have suggested a testis transplant in place of an undiscovered anatomical dysfunction, although a new testis was useless.

Much later--in 1983 to be exact--the Brit Giles Brindley, a former athlete and now a urologist, demonstrated the result of years of experimentation by injecting his penis with a substance [phenoxybenzamine] prior to giving a speech on potency, the crucial moment being when he dropped his trousers to show his erection to the conference of urologists. The problem was thusly vanquished--in that men could now have erections thanks to phenoxybenzamine being injected directly into their penis--until Pfizer came out with a little blue tablet, Viagra, in 1998, the fastest selling pill in world history, earning the company billions, the users in the unknown millions because the pills are offered by the Net, more prized and hush-hushed than cocaine--making the stockholders filthy rich.

THE PHALLUS IN ANCIENT GREECE AND ROME
Antonie van Leeuwenhjoek
Paracelsus
Maypoles
Priapus
Pan

All historical sources conclude that the Romans couldn't care less if a man stuck his dick in a girl or a boy: it just didn't matter. Caesar himself was known to be a man to every woman, a woman to every man. His soldiers sang ditties to that effect as they marched along, perhaps not always to Caesar's amusement; in fact, Caesar was far more sensitive about losing his hair than having lost his cherry, when young, to King Nicomedes who happened to have been a Bithynian like Antinous, and like Antinous Nicomedes was noted for the dimensions of his member. The words hetero and homo didn't exist yet because the distinction between them was immaterial.

Whereas Greek boys were encouraged to have older lovers and to learn from them, the Romans had sex for pleasure as long as the participants respected two iron-clad principles [although, as we all well know, all iron-clad principles are made to be disregarded]: A Roman male could not have sex with another Roman male. If he was horny and a slave [or a foreigner or anyone else, as long as he/she wasn't a Roman] passed by, he/she was fair game. The second principle was that a Roman male had to do the penetrating. It was he who was *vir*ile [*vir* meaning man in Latin]. A corollary to the two principles was the very strong preference for young smooth hairless bodies, often between the ages of 14 and 20, marked by the onset of down on the boy's cheeks (permissible too on his butt cheeks). Greek boys had Greek lovers, often many, from whom the boys gained the key to life: *knowledge*. The boys were normally passive, the men active, and when the boys became men, the roles were inversed: they took on a boy of their own, their belovèd, and they became the boy's lover and teacher. There was also a practical side to Greek love. A lover would never ever show weakness before his belovèd and vice versa, which made them the fiercest fighting force the world has ever known.

The Romans and Greeks practiced vaginal and anal penetration, intercrural insertion and fellatio. Mutual masturbation and circle jerks were rarely mentioned because they were so common between schoolboys, a little like boys pissing together. Parents despaired of keeping their sons, if they were beautiful, chaste. Roman boys did have access to slaves, just like their elders did, on whom they could practice intercourse, intercrural or anal. Diogenes the Cynic says that of the three appetites, food, drink and sex, sex is the easiest to fulfill as one need only rub oneself to obtain instant satisfaction.

Sex was found in brothels and latrines and taverns, parks and gardens and any other place sheltered from public view. Hadrian's successor, Emperor Lucius Verus, opened a tavern in his own home in order to create a climate for debauch. Male prostitutes showed their wares in parks and gardens then, as they do today along certain roads encompassing Rome, where lads bear all to passing motorists, just like boys did to passers-by in antiquity, from Antioch to the City of the Seven Hills. Many rent boys turned to acting to supplement their incomes, as did Hadrian's favorite Pylades.

Since just being a wife was enough status for most women, men were free to look elsewhere for pleasure. In Rome love was always in the air [just like today]. The Romans had adopted many of the Greek gods and their myths, especially those which dealt with Apollo and Hyacinth, Hercules and Hylas, Achilles and Patroclus, Zeus and his cupbearer and bedmate Ganymede. Antinous's role was strikingly similar to that played by Ganymede, and as he was Greek he was a safe foreigner, although it's doubtful that Hadrian would have turned him away should he have been a Roman citizen. The Greeks were not obliged to look for sex in gardens or taverns or back alleys. They had gymnasiums where they could openly entice boys, although not those under age 18. Rich parents sent slaves to accompany their sons to and from the gym. Sex between boys was so current that we have the story of the Greek boy who didn't share his schoolmates' interest in men. He prayed to Zeus so that he too could be moved by the love of boys, but when this failed to happen, he committed suicide.

At age 15 Caesar exchanged the *toga praetexta* with its purple fringe for the pure white *toga virilis*. He was now a recognized citizen of Rome, responsible, in case of his father's death, for his mother and sisters and younger brothers. In Caesar's case, he had become the paterfamilias. He also put aside his *bulla praetexta*, a charm of gold held in a leather sack that parents put around their boy's neck, at age 9 days [time to see if he lived through the unsanitary conditions of childbirth], aimed at warding off evil spirits. The bulla, along with a lock of the boy's hair or, if the boy could, the first shavings from his chin, were placed on the family altar and dedicated to the Lares, guardian deities of the household. Mothers recuperated the bulla to protect the boy as he grew, to protect him especially from envious people who might wish him harm. The ceremony of the Lares must have been very moving and certainly would be today if it existed [in its place some nations cut off a boy's prepuce, disfiguring him for life, depriving him of what should be his own choice when he reaches the age of reason]. The ceremony took place on the 17th of March. Forty-four years later, nearly to the day, Caesar would be assassinated by men who had worshipped him until then, one of whom could have *conceivably* been his son, as Brutus was born when Caesar was nearly 16, and Brutus's mother was a very long-term mistress of Caesar's.

A boy's bulla enclosed an erect phallus which was to protect him from being ruined by the introduction of a phallus into his anus, the absolute opposite of what the Greeks were doing, even if a Roman boy could have anal sex with another non-citizen boy or man. In fact, many virtues were passed from a Greek man to a Greek boy when the man ejaculated within him, as he implanted his *arête* into the boy--*arête* being courage, wisdom and honesty. It was the reason for the cult of Harmodius, the lover, and Aristogeiton, his belovèd, as we see in this story:

Hippias and Hipparchus were joint dictators in Athens. Hipparchus fancied the wondrous Harmodius who refused his advances. To gain revenge, Hipparchus refused to let Harmodius's sister take part in the Panathenaea Games, accusing her of not being a virgin, a requirement. Harmodius and his lover Aristogeiton decided to rid Athens of the dictatorship and thusly redeem the honor of Harmodius's sister. With daggers hidden in their chitons, the boys fell on Hipparchus at the foot of the Acropolis, stabbing him to death. Hipparchus's guards immediately killed Harmodius, and Aristogeiton was captured. While being tortured to reveal any coconspirators, Aristogeiton agreed to tell the truth if Hippias would promise him clemency, sealed with a handshake. When Hippias complied, Aristogeiton laughed at his having shaken the hand of his own brother's murderer. Hippias, mad with fury, thrust his dagger into Aristogeiton's throat.

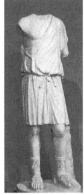

A boy's chiton.

After the death of his brother, Hippias set up a more drastic form of dictatorship, becoming very unpopular. Harmodius and Aristogeiton were declared liberators and countless statues were raised in their names. One statue was later captured by Xerxes who took it to Susa where Alexander the Great found it and returned it to Athens where it received divine honors. The legend of the two boys, and the sanctity of their love, was of such importance that even in Roman times statues of them continued to be sculpted. Their ancestors received vast privileges, such as free meals and front-row theater seats.

But a Roman boy's own anus was to remain virgin, his *vir*--his virility--depended on it. The penis *glans* comes from Latin and had exactly the same meaning for the Romans as it does for us, with the addition that it was also the word for bullet, the word for the projectiles shot from slings, and they could be inscribed as bombs dropped over Germany had been--in Marc Antony's war against Octavius his bullets had written descriptions on how his men would penetrate Octavius's ass. Both Greeks and Romans had a fascination for the phallus, and it was portrayed on walls in homes in order to bring good luck and ward off evil, as seen in Pompeii [one wall showing un erect phallus and two testicles read: *Hic Habitat Felicitas*, Here Resides Happiness--another example of phallic obsession]. Paintings of phalluses were a common sight in the baths, pictures in differing degrees of tumescence, always a pleasurable reminder of what awaited the bathers in the afternoon or night. The phallus has been represented in amulets and on cave walls for 30,000 years.

Because Priapus had a huge member he was less appreciated in Greece, for reasons explained elsewhere, than in Rome.

Statues of Hermes, god of travelers, were erected at crossroads. Their particularity was a fully engorged phallus with ample foreskin. As crossroads were places of encounter, the phalli took on erotic signification. Boys looking for adventure would stroke them for luck, girls searching for husbands did likewise, and women wanting children made pilgrimages to the sites--in fact, the phalli were polished to a luster. During the night preceding an expedition to capture Sicily, Hermes's phalli throughout Athens were vandalized, most probably by drunken pranksters, exactly the milieu frequented--and most often led--by Alcibiades, a youth known by all for his brilliant intellect and total absence of morality. As during our own times, in ancient Athens too people were unduly respectful of those of high birth and affluence, the reason they were reluctant to attack Alcibiades head on. The destruction was also heresy, as Hermes was an Olympian god. And it was the worst possible omen prior to a military enterprise. But there was a strong possibility that Alcibiades would escape punishment thanks to his connection with Pericles and his immense wealth (19).

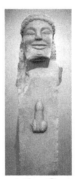

Hermes at the Crossroads.

The problem with Sicily began in 415 B.C.--the 17th year of the Peloponnesian war--when a delegation from the island came to tell Athenians that the time was ripe for them to conquer Syracuse, the most important city-state on Sicily. The people of Syracuse were ethnical Dorians, as were the Spartans, whereas the members of the delegation from the much smaller city-state of Segesta were ethnical Ionians, as were the Athenians. Syracuse, the island's principal city, was about the size of Athens. It was rich and the island richer. Its capture would supply Athens with immense wealth, resources and more wheat than Athens would ever need. Sicily was the breadbasket of the Greek world, as, later, Egypt would be for the Romans.

Alcibiades wanted to go to war and soon he had the Athenians on their knees, drawing sketches of the island in the sand, each vying to place the major island towns in their right places. Men and boys were forming lines to join up as members of the expedition, certain that they would reap gold through sacking the palaces and homes of the rich inhabitants. The delegation from Segesta arrived with 60 talents of silver (a talent weighed 26 kilos) and plates of solid gold. In addition, they declared that their temples and citizens possessed a treasure in solid gold vessels. The Athenians sent a delegation to assure itself that this was so; the members returned with smiles on their faces. This turned the heads of the Athenians, and especially that of the handsome Alcibiades who was always in need of lucre.

When the Athenian noble Nicias saw that Alcibiades had stirred up the blood of Athenians hungry for war and the riches reaped through war, he threw in his support, so long as he was named general and the size of the fleet and the number of warriors involved in Alcibiades' plan were at the very least doubled, thereby giving Athens a chance at success. He did warn his friends, however, to beware of Alcibiades who would one day endanger Athens in order to live a brilliant life of his own.

When the full Athenian force did finally arrive in Sicily, it discovered that the solid gold brought to Athens by the Segestaeans was only silver plated with gold, and the solid gold vessels the expedition had seen at Segesta had only been the same vessels passed from house to house and from temple to temple!

Alcibiades wanted to be judged for the crime against Hermes before setting sail for Sicily, aware that during his absence his enemies, were he not judged, would do what was necessary to turn heads and buy votes. After all, the penalty for heresy was death. Athenians were as serious about offending the gods as were Europeans, later, under the Inquisition. Had his request to be judged before setting sail been accepted, he would have certainly been acquitted for the simple reason that the Athenians needed him for their intervention. But the request was refused, and he prepared to leave for Sicily as co-general with Nicias at the head of what Thucydides said was the greatest armada ever raised by a single Greek state, 134 triremes and a far greater number of smaller ships, as well as 30,000 men. Diodorus Siculus recounts that all of Athens--inhabitants, friends, lovers and children--traipsed behind the warriors as they made their way to the Piraeus, singing and waving fronds. The ships bobbing in the harbor had been fully decked out with banners, flags and pennants, their sides covered with the shields of all the participating countries, those furnishing soldiers or money. Perfume burners and fires in bronze vessels consumed incense in such quantity that the air was misty with it. Lovers kissed their friends goodbye and the boys went off to their fates

Just after arrival at the island of Sicily, a ship, the *Salaminia*, came from Athens demanding that Alcibiades return to stand trial for the destruction of the Hermes's statues. Judging from the behavior of the emissaries sent to bring him back, Alcibiades knew what awaited him at home. He knew that the Athenians had perfected the art of using men for their own benefit, but that they would then humble and chasten them when the men became too powerful or too well known. This was a highly dangerous move on the part of the Athenians because the army and sailors favored Alcibiades, who had an uncanny way of winning over the men under his command; the Athenians therefore treated him with kid gloves, promising anything to get him aboard. Otherwise, they knew, the whole army would mutiny. Besides the army's love for him, the soldiers also felt that under someone indecisive like Nicias the war could drag on for an eternity, with no riches, as Alcibiades had promised, at the end. Alcibiades agreed to return but on his own ship.

Unknown to all, his true destination was Sparta. A Spartan nurse had cared for Alcibiades and had instilled the love of Sparta in the child's heart. Also, his family had had traditional connections with Sparta. When a Spartan delegation came to Athens in search of a peace agreement in 421 Alcibiades, thanks to his family, enjoyed privileged access to the ephors. Alcibiades didn't waste time in seducing the Spartans. He wore their coarse clothes, bathed in cold water, ate their disgusting broths, drank their inferior wines, and bedded their women, one of whom was King Agis' wife who bore Alcibiades' son Leotychides. Alcibiades counted on Leotychides to found a new Spartan race of Alcibiadesian origin. It didn't help matters much when Agis' wife went around calling her baby Alcibiades, the name she preferred to Leotychides. Alcibiades could play the role of the perfect Spartan, Plutarch tells us, because he was the perfect chameleon--all things to all men, displaying virtue or vice as the occasion called. It must have been marvelous to observe his technique because men really liked and appreciated him, and being a man's man is not an easy task. Plutarch goes on to say that in Sparta he devoted himself to athletic exercises; in Ionia he enjoyed the luxury of the baths, oiled and perfumed, at ease with the fondling of both sexes; in Thrace he drank to the dregs among the dregs; in Thessaly he awed all with his horsemanship; and in Persia he exceeded even the Persians in magnificence. He was thusly accused of playing a double game, but men have been known to willfully march to more than just one tune without having treacherous motives. [The rest of the story can be found in my book *Alcibiades*.]

The Liberalia was a hugely important stage in a boy's life, when he discarded the toga praetexta for the toga virilis, or man's garment. As boys reached their puberty far later than today, the festival took place when the lad was 14 to 16, and as the festival's god, Liber Pater, represented the reproductive seed, the ceremony followed the boy's first ejaculation. At the same time the boys exchanged one robe for another, they took off the charm of gold and leather they had worn around their necks up to then, the bulla praetexta, that they placed on an altar, accompanied by a sprig of their hair and/or shaved chin whiskers if they had grown any. The bulla praetexta was recuperated by mothers and kept to ward off evil, as said, its purpose during the lad's childhood.

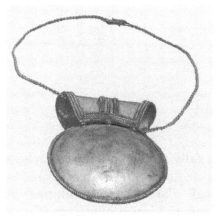

bulla praetexta

We don't know how the boys proved they could ejaculate, probably doing so in front of friends, or perhaps everyone took his word for it.

Liber Pater was more ancient than Bacchus, and was the Roman version of the Greek god Dionysus.

Greeks and Romans sprinkled semen over their crops to assure their growth. Paracelsus, introduced in a moment, wrote that a man could produce a child without a woman if his semen was placed in a glass jar with horse-dung for forty days, after which it had to be nourished for forty weeks with a man's blood. ''It will become a true and living infant,'' promised Paracelsus.

For Aristotle what counted was semen, the woman being a mere incubator, while Apollo said a woman was a furrow where a man's seed was thrust, the true parent being he who plants the seed, not the woman who only tends it. Such a belief that semen sufficed to make humans was reinforced by Zeus who gave birth to Athena through his head and Dionysus through his thigh.

For Aristotle semen was produced in both the brain and the spinal column, transmitted to the testicles, the one on the right, being perfect, produced boys, the one on the left, incomplete, girls. Da Vinci too, despite his days of dissection and extreme interest in male genitalia, believed that semen came through the spinal column, by way of an inexistent seminal channel.

All life issued from an egg, said Aristotle, and eggs issued from coagulated semen. The Dutchman Antonie van Leeuwenhjoek was the first to see semen under a microscope, in 1678, and believed that each spermatozoa was a fully-formed human.

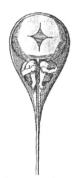

The fully-formed human in each spermatozoa.

The man called Paracelsus [Philippus Aureolus Theophrastus Bombastus von Hohenheim] was a physician often compared to Luther, his contemporary, because Luther protested against the wrongs of the Catholic church, while Paracelsus protested against the wrongs of medicine as practiced then.

What interests us specifically here was Paracelsus's attempt to resurrect himself by having his phallus cut off on his deathbed and buried in manure drenched in blood. The attempt failed when his servant opened the grave too late to find the baby, and came upon the remains that had turned to dust. Now, if the reader doubts the veracity of such a resurrection, I'd like to draw his attention to a similar attempt, this one successful, that we find in this extract from my book *TROY*, one involving Zeus and his favorite son, Hermes:

"Uh, where was I? Ah, yes. So Hermes and I stopped at some peasant's hovel and to our astonishment we were hospitably offered warm wine and vittles. To thank the old man, Hermes and I asked him to confide his heart's innermost wish. The poor old fellow sighed and said that although he was impotent and his wife long dead, his heart's desire was to have a son.

"Now, I would have instructed him to eat a certain potent mushroom that has wondrous regenerative powers and then get himself a mistress. But not Hermes. After some thought he told the old man to go to his wife's grave and take out her bones. He was then to sacrifice a bull to Almighty Myself, skin the hide into which he would place his wife's bones, piss on the remains, and bury the hide and its contents in his wife's grave. At the end of nine months he was to return and dig it all up.

"The old man did as instructed, and when he returned nine months later he found a boy at the bottom of the pit, swaddled in the old hide. We named him 'Orion', meaning 'He-Who-Makes-Water' in Greek, giving us today's word urine."

Back to Paracelsus. He was both peculiar and ahead of his times. Born in Switzerland in 1493, he was among other things a chemist who invented the word zinc, and a medical doctor trained by his chemist and physician father. He was a military surgeon in Venice. He held the chair of medicine at the University of Basil and founded the chair of medicine at the University of Leipzig, where he officially adopted the name Paracelsus, ''surpassing Celsus'', the Greek philosopher. Although he ranted against how medicine was being practiced at the time, as an astrologist he believed in astrological talismans for curing diseases. He believed that sulpher, mercury and salt were causes of all diseases, and by altering them one could cure a patient. Good health came through the balance of bodily minerals. Plants that resembled a body part were capable of curing that part. Stars were vehicles for poisoning the body, but also for curing it, so if a bad star infected a part of the body it had to be found and neutralized by a good star. As everything in the universe was interconnected, herbs, minerals and chemicals could be put at the service of good health. He was the first to advocate cleanliness in the treatment of wounds and sought to impose mercury as a cure for syphilis. He recommended iron in the strengthening of poor blood and discovered Alpine water during his travels and recommended its curative powers. Finally, he believed that the mentally ill were not possessed by evil spirits and should be treated humanly.

Romans wore phallic amulets, *fascina*, to enhanced their sexual potency as well as to protect them against harm, *fascina* from which we draw our word fascinating. Roman soldiers and generals wore amulets with phalluses for luck before battle, and anyone else, in need of luck, wore them at any time.

The Greeks had Heracles and his phallic club, Zeus his thunderbolts and Poseidon his trident, all symbols of the potency and power of the phallus. Later, some villages in England dressed maypoles, phallic symbols that Cromwell forbad as a symbol of ''superstition and wickedness.''

It was because Christianity prohibited one from honoring the phallus that the maypole came into existence, the site of weddings and, like the Hermes phalli, places girls could go to discreetly touch it, in the hope it would bring her luck in finding a boy and becoming pregnant if she had one, *and* she would return and stroke it again so that her baby would have the scepter every man desired in the first born.

Believed by Freud to have had its origin as a pagan phallus symbol, and believed by most people today to represent the male phallus, its real origin, lost in time, may have been something entirely sexually innocent. That said, everything in that form is taken as being phallic, masts of ships, the Washington Monument, minarets, the royal scepter, *et al*, which is proof again that we have only that on the brain, adolescent boys apparently thinking about "it" or doing "it" every ten minutes of the day, maintain some psychologists. Today maypoles are raised throughout the world, to the glee of boys and girls who dance at their feet, welcoming in spring, *the* season of love.

The view of the scepter was often a question of life or death in ancient times, when a newborn was laid at the feet of a man and the blanket opened to reveal the sex. If it was a boy the man would take it up and hold it over his head, if a girl, and he wished to recognize it, he would say, "Let it eat!" If not the child was exposed outside, perhaps saved by a passing farmer who took her home to be raised for work in the fields and to fulfill his sexual needs.

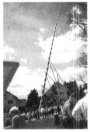

Raising a maypole near Munich.

In our own time boys playing guitars is recognized as subliminal public masturbation [and in some concerts they are played by boys who are totally naked or wear socks covering their dicks]. Freud agreed that a cigar was phallic and implied fellatio, but stated that it was also "just a cigar".

Priapus

The reader may remember that when Aphrodite lay under Ares, both entrapped in Hephaestus's net, she heard Dionysus praise her beauty, and promised herself they would later meet and mate, the product of which union was Priapus. Hera made him foul-mouthed and ugly to avenge herself on Aphrodite who persuaded Paris to award her the Golden Apple, and she made sure that he was rejected by the Olympians. He found shelter with shepherds who appreciated his ribald humor and ever-erect phallus, and was especially honored in Bithynia where all Bithynian boys are hugely hung, one of the reasons Emperor Hadrian was mad about Antinous, a Bithynian (7).

A minor god in Greece, he was of great importance in Rome where he was worn around the neck in a good-luck amulet, and was pictured on walls as a source of fortune and fertility, and of course every lad aspired to possess a bit of his ever-erect virility and lustiness. Placed at crossroad, in gardens and doorways for the reasons cited above, he was also a warning to thieves that they would be anally assaulted should they enter the premises, that or Priapus would bludgeon them with his weighty endowment.

Priapus was also the protector of sailors, and encouraged their randy pursuits, for which they are renowned even today.

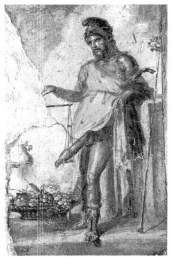

A fresco from the Casa dei Vettii, Pompeii, depicting Priapus weighing his phallus against a bag of gold. Unlike the Greeks, ancient Romans admired huge members, applauded them in the baths, and had a sense of humor in portraying them.

The cult of Priapus surpassed that of Pan and replaced the phallic deity of the Etruscans. Phalli everywhere brought luck and assured fertility, while protecting the wearer of phallic amulets from the evil eye.

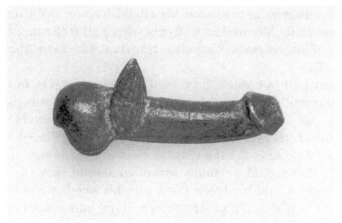

A phallic amulet, often shown with wings.

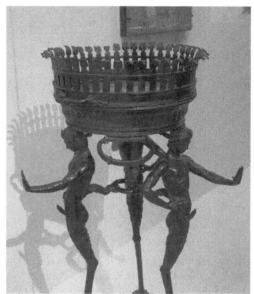

Three priapic satyrs from a tripod found in Herculaneum.

In a Roman household there was a statue of Priapus, on whose erection a Roman woman put a garland, one for each time her husband had ''honored'' her the night before. Messalina purportedly placed 14 garlands on the phallus following a night with 14 athletes.

Pan

God of the wild and shepherds, he has the legs and horns of a goat, as do fauns and satyrs, and because he lives in the wilds--forests, groves and woods--he is connected to fertility. Son of Hermes and a nymph, Arcadia was the seat of his worship. Doted with great sexual powers, his phallus is huge, and his father, Hermes, taught him its use through autoeroticism, which Pan then taught to shepherds. While some claim that the Great God Pan died, killed by Christianity, it is only a rumor, and false at that, as Pan shall live on as long as shepherds take pleasure in pleasuring themselves.

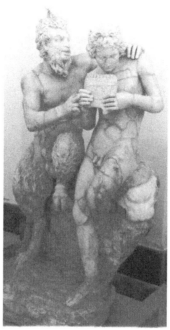

Pan seducing Daphnis.

CHRISTIANITY / THE ERECT CHRIST / OATH GIVING

''There is probably no religion in which a substratum of the phallic cult does not exist,'' writes Alain Doniélou who translated the *Kama Sutra* [the original translation of the *Kama Sutra* was by Richard Francis Burton, explorer and homosexual (2)]. The Christian cross, as an example, is an upright phallus with testicles on both sides.

Because of the existence of Pope Joan, an Englishwoman, the *sedia stercoraria* was invented, a chair with a hole that newly-elected popes were obliged to sit on while a cardinal checked him out from underneath. What is incredible in the story of Pope Joan is that even now we do not know if she existed or not, despite the Vatican's attempt to ridicule her reign, calling it a legend [which it may well be].

Joan supposedly disguised herself as a man so she could be near her lover, perhaps a priest or a cardinal, and as she had great ability she rose through church hierarchy to become pope. She was found out during a procession in the midst of which she gave birth, a place apparently avoided by Vatican processions to this day. She was then murdered [one version has her being immediately tied to a horse's tail and dragged through Rome, stoned by passers-by until dead]. She was first mentioned in a chronicle written by Jean de Mailly in 1250. She supposedly reigned somewhere during the 800s, and was accepted as having existed until the question of how it was possible that a woman could have headed the church came up in the 16th century.

The *sedia stercoraria* was thusly constructed, which permitted an aspiring pope's testicles to freely hang while someone checked through a curtain behind, exclaiming, *''Duos habet et bene pendentes,''* he has two and they dangle nicely. This too is now said to be a legend, and the chair previously shown to visitors is now said to have been one used at the time, even publicly by Louis XIV, to do his business [the contents scrupulously studied to make sure they consisted of the correct humors].

Freshly baptized Emperor Charlemagne crowned Pope Leo III and offered him the true prepuce of Christ, one of a purported 18 to have existed during the Middle Ages, one of which was sent to Antwerp by King Baldwin I of Jerusalem during the First Crusade. During the Renaissance Dutch and German artists portrayed Jesus with an erection, that some said, later, was proof of Christ risen.

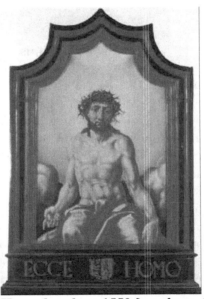

Maerten Jocobsz van Heemskerck, c. 1550 [you have to look very closely to spot the erection].

In biblical times one testified by touching the penis or cupping the testicles or grasping the entire genitalia, the word testify, itself, coming from *testis* "to witness", itself from testes.

Abraham ordered a servant to swear by the Lord, all the while palming Abraham's balls.

When the time came for Israel to die he made Joseph "put his hand under my thigh" [biblical speak for testicles], and promise Israel that he would not be buried in Egypt.

When Arabs, today, swear an oath they do so by stroking their penises through the fabric of their clothing, and I've seen Mediterranean men touch themselves when emphasizing the veracity of what they were saying. [Arabs, by the way, claim that there are three insatiables: the desert, the grave and a woman's vulva.]

The church allowed thousands of boys to be castrated so that church ceremonies could be accompanied by the exquisite purity found only in pre-puberty boy choirs. Only boys who had been castrated by accident were allowed, but the church fathers knew that it was an industry, one that caused the loss of hundreds of lives when done in unclean conditions. In the same way, the Roman church has allowed thousands and thousands of lads to be abused by priests, the only mystery being how the parents of boys continue to honor a religion responsible for such filth. [Tut-tut.]

THE PHALLUS IN RENAISSANCE ART

Roman artists were inspired by Greek art in all things, down to the modest size of the penis, the Greeks who believed, as said elsewhere, that big phalluses were possessed by ugly, uncivilized lowlifes, while for Romans they represented virility. The Renaissance was the rebirth of Greek culture, and so Michelangelo followed the Greek custom of showing the male endowment smaller than was the case for Roman men, while several historians suggest that *David*, preparing to combat against Goliath, was demonstrating his concern about the coming battle in two ways, his deeply furrowed brow, and his genitals, the shrinking of which occur in time of stress.

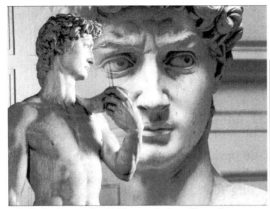
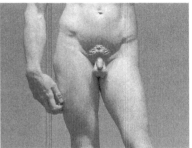

Michelangelo followed the Greek custom of the small penis, here his *David,* and below the *Victorious Youth* and the *Kritios Boy.*

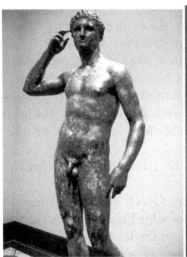
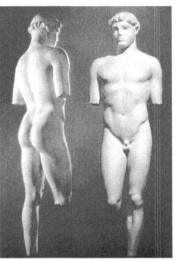

MASACCIO
1401 – 1428

For a boy to die at age 26 is a tragedy and, alas, we don't know why although many perished from malaria and the plague, and in this case the great biographer Vasari claims he was poisoned by a jealous competitor. His first name was Tommaso, the shortened version of which is Maso, meaning messy; Massacio is said to be a comical version of Maso. Added to this was his quasi life-long friendship with Masolino (Little Tom), an older man with whom he traveled to Rome and worked so inseparably that they were known as "the duo". That they were lover and belovèd is unknown but highly likely given the mores in the ateliers and the sexuality of the times.

Masaccio lost his father at age 5 and gained a brother that same year, Giovanni called *Lo Scheggia*, the splinter, himself a painter. Masaccio was probably apprenticed at age 12. His and his friends' works are thought to have greatly influenced Michelangelo.

So little is known about Masaccio and Masolino's paintings that some are thought to have been left unfinished, while others believe the ''unfinished'' parts are in reality those damaged for one reason or another. Filippino Lippi is thought to have finished some of the paintings, while others believe Lippi just restored certain segments.

Masaccio was one of the first painters to use linear perspective, perhaps aided by Brunelleschi. Marble was automatically three-dimensional while a painter was obliged to create depth on a flat surface. Masaccio mastered the three-dimensional concept, and how to create illusion. He understood depth through perspective and through the gradations of colors.

On the painting of the *Holy Trinity* in the church Santa Maria Novella in Florence, above the skeleton, we find the famous inscription: ''I once was what you are; what I am you shall be.''

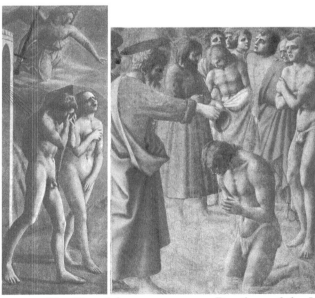

The Expulsion   *Baptism of the Neophytes*

POLLAIOLO
1429 – 1498

Antonio del Pollaiolo (1429 – 1498) worked with his brother Piero (1443 – 1496), both born in Florence, both named after their father's trade, poultry, whose works are often confounded, although Antonio is the most accomplished of the two. Both studied painting under Andrea del Castagno but Antonio specialized in metal work and engraving, the most celebrated of which is his *Battle of the Nude Men*, five with headbands and five without, fighting in pairs.

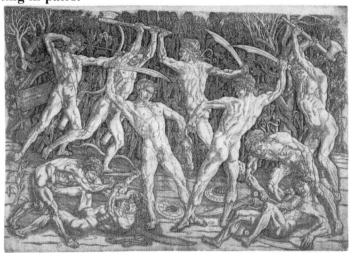

Battle of the Nude Men

Both brothers were born in Florence and worked in Rome where Antonio sculpted the tombs of two popes, Sixtus IV and Innocent VIII, found today in St. Peter's. Both had their own tombs, together, at the church of San Pietro in Vincoli.

The male forms in their paintings are anatomically correct as both excelled in human dissection. Their best works were said to be combined efforts, notably their *Heracles and Antaeus* in bronze and the painting *St. Sebastian*. Both show muscles placed with anatomical perfection thanks to his assiduous dissections.

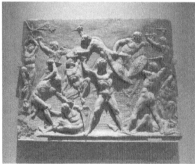

Males nudes in combat

MANTEGNA
1431 – 1506

The workshop of Francesco Squarcione, in Padua, was extremely successful, and those who found a place there, nearly 150--Uccello, Filippo Lippi, Donatello, etc.--were lucky, as Squarcione, a former tailor, was passionately moved by humanism and Greek art, traveling the breadth of Italy and Greece to collect antique statues and vases. His collection was open to all, especially to those who wished to do drawings of the artifacts. But more than his collection and his other apprentices, it was Mantegna his preferred student, whom he later adopted. Mantegna's masterpiece is said to have been the frescoes of Sant'Agostino degli Eremitani, most of which were bombed into fragments in 1944.

He executed his first *St. Sebastian* in Padua, perhaps in thanks for his having survived the plague. A rider with a scythe is present in the upper left corner of the clouds, but one must look very hard to make it out:

It seems that Mantegna's style, the portrayal of rocks and marble, the rigidity of forms, the bony muscularity, came through Squarcione and his collection, of which Mantegna did countless studies. But he was also influenced by the Bellini, a Venetian family of artists, pioneers in oil paintings. He married Jacopo Bellini's daughter Nicolosia, but as the Bellini were rivals of Squarcione, and Mantegna had not gained Squarcione's permission to marry, they became enemies.

Mantegna went to Mantua to became court artist to Ludovico III Gonzaga who paid him a princely sum because he was the first artist that the extremely artistic Gonzaga had allured. Mantegna built a mansion and filled it with art, but shortly afterwards suffered the loss of his son Bernardino.

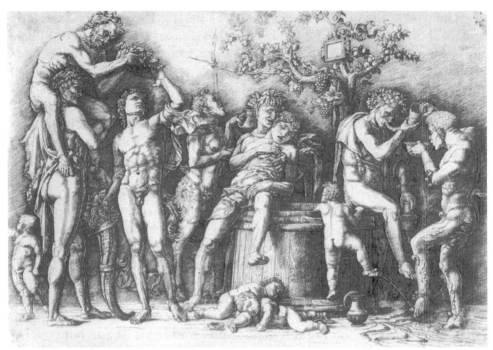

Bacchanal with Wine

Called to Rome by Innocent VIII, he did frescos later destroyed by Pius VI to make way for other paintings. It was in Rome that Mantegna met Djem Sultan who had gained the capital after losing a battle fought with his brother over who would become sultan. Djem had first gone to Rhodes where the Knights Hospitaler kept him prisoner in exchange for gold from the new sultan. In Rome Innocent tried to convert him to Christianity and to use him to mount a crusade against his own people, both without success. The sultan paid the pope 120,000 crowns to keep Djem in luxurious imprisonment, at the time a sum equal to the entire yearly papal revenues. Enlisted by Charles VIII to help capture Naples, Djem died of fever (although others claim he was poisoned became his brother stopped payments for his care). The Ottomans wanted his body back for decent burial and succeeded four years later, when they'd offered enough gold. As Rome could not match the freedom and friendship he had known in Mantua, Mantegna returned there where he painted nine tempera pictures known as the *Triumphs of Caesar*, his existing *chef d'oeuvre*, now in Hampton Court, England.

His wife died and in his 70s he fathered a son, Giovanni Andrea. After his death Giovanni and other sons he had had built a beautiful monument in his honor in the church Sant'Andrea.

On the lower right-hand corner of his last *Sebastian* one sees an extinguished candle with a banner that reads: Nothing is stable that is not divine. Vasari finishes his life of Mantegna by saying that a kinder, more gentle man never existed.

SIGNORELLI
1445 – 1523

The importance of the nude form during the Renaissance is an absolute mystery to me. Naturally, with the rebirth of philosophy and literature came the resurgence of the naked body so wonderfully shown through the digging up of the *Laocoön*, the end-all of homoerotic sculpture [and the cover sculpture of my book *TROY*]. But this was for the intelligentsia who had their own pornography thanks to Giulio Romano and private collections like that in the possession of Charles VIII of France. But for the people, totally illiterate for the most part, paintings were biblical lessons into the content of the Bible, whose inhabitants were clothed. Yet here we have Signorelli's anatomically perfect full-frontal nudes in every form of action [other than sexual, for which we have Romano--although Romano's sexually explicit etchings were in private hands only]. Signorelli's nudes not only got through church censorship, Vasari claims that Signorelli was *the* most popular artist of his times. A second conundrum is how the church allowed dissections which not even the Romans and the medically-attuned Arabs permitted. The University of Bologna was said to have practiced *public* dissections for centuries.

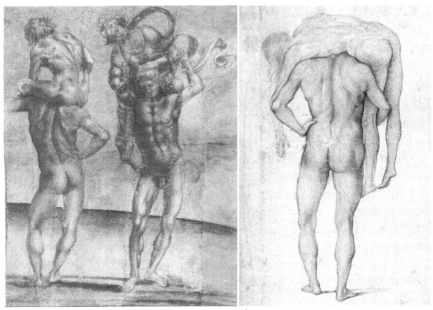

Drawings

Fewer people took more advantage of dissections than Signorelli, da Vinci and Michelangelo. Signorelli was born and buried in Cortona. He invented, says Vasari, ''a world of fanciful extravagances, demons, antichrists, devils, hell fires, all Dantesque, all totally naked and totally alive''. When very young, Signorelli was taken in by Vasari's own great-grandfather, Lazzaro Vasari. The rest of his life is a mystery, as Vasari dedicates only six short pages to him, and then only to describe his paintings, although he does tell us that one of Signorelli's works was restored by Il Sodoma who ruined it, and, wonders Vasari, ''Where do people of little talent'' ... like Sodoma ... ''get off restoring the works of geniuses?''

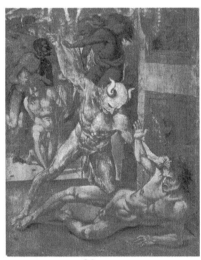

Charon

We do learn that while Signorelli was painting a Christ his beloved son ''handsome in face and body,'' says Vasari, was killed. [Vasari appreciated male beauty and deeply scratched the back of a boy Cellini offered him for the night, without paying the boy for the sex and for the cuts that had drawn blood.] Signorelli ''had him stripped naked and painted him, so that he would always have a portrait of his boy at hand''. He also painted the face of Christ in his son's image.

Signorelli was one of many called to Rome by Julius II and then summarily replaced by Raphael. Vasari goes on to say that there was not a man more courteous, sincere and friendly than Signorelli, thanks to which he had a never-ending stream of students, and held the most important positions in the governing of Cortona. He died at around age 82.

DA VINCI
1452-1519

Leonardo was gorgeous and so were his boys, beginning with Salaì, magnificent in da Vinci's two paintings, *St. John the Baptist* and *Bacchus*, the absolute ultimate in homoerotic art. The beauty of Leonardo can be admired in Francesco Botticini's *Tobias and the Three Archangels*, Leonardo shown as the first angel; and Verrocchio's *Archangel Michael*.

Salaì was Leonardo's nickname for his boy lover, meaning Little Devil, bestowed when Salaì, unmanageable and stubborn, hotheaded and careless, proved to be a liar and a not-so-accomplished--although highly assiduous-- thief. This at the prepubescent age of ten. A very close friend of Leonardo's, Giacomo Andrea, was present during one of the first meals shared with Salaì. It is suspected that Leonardo's idea for the *Vitruvian Man,* the male body made up of two superimposed figures showing four arms and four legs, was originally Andrea's invention, and bares an amazing resemblance to Leonardo himself. Of Salaì Andrea said he was a glutton who ate as much as four monks, spilled the wine and broke whatever his fingers came upon. Another friend, the painter, architect, writer and historian Giorgio Vasari wrote that Salaì was ''a graceful and beautiful boy with curly hair and a delight to Leonardo.'' There is no doubt that he was Leonardo's bedmate, the only question being from what age? Along the line Leonardo drew him with a huge erection, a drawing called *The Incarnate Angel.* But Salaì was such a trickster that he may have drawn in the phallus himself on one of his master's many drawings of him. (Another drawing is entitled *Salaì's Ass,* the boy's buttocks shown surrounded by penises.)

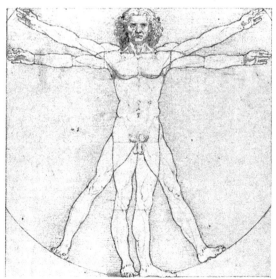

The Vitruvian Man

Numerous times Salaì made off with Leonardo's money, but as the painter had endless commissions, he was rich and, at the end of his life, even wealthy. Salaì is said to have bought clothes with most of the lucre he swiped, at one point possessing thirty pairs of shoes. Throughout his entire life he remained by Leonardo's side, at times replaced, as with the handsome Melzi. Melzi to whom Leonardo left half of his fortune, the other half going to Salaì. But most importantly, both boys remained loyal to the master, both present at his side to witness his last breath.

Da Vinci's *John the Baptist* is the most beautiful portrait of a young man that has ever been put on canvas. He kept it and the *Mona Lisa* until the very end, at the Chateau of Clos Lucé, a chateau given to him by François I, who is believed to have held his head as he expired, perhaps da Vinci's last gaze on Salaì at his bedside or Salaì, much younger, the model for *John the Baptist*.

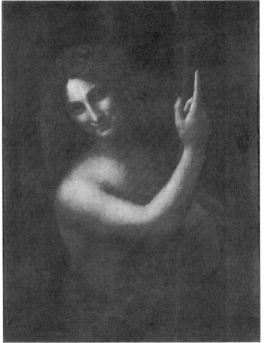

John the Baptist

No one will ever know why the child Salaì was chosen by Leonardo. Leonardo himself said he had come upon him while the child was drawing, and seeing potential, he made enquiries into his family. Finding them poor, he made them an offer they couldn't refuse. Leonardo was thirty-eight, an age when a man begins to think of settling down, tired of running after boys his ever-so-slightly decline in beauty was more and more compensated for by a few easy coins, of which, for him, there was no dearth. Already, at age twenty-four, he'd been arrested by the Florentine Office of the Night, he and a gang of his friends, all accused of sodomy. He got off as the charge was difficult to prove, but it shows that, like other Florentines, he was no parvenu to male-to-male intercourse. His interest for those of his own sex was already well known, as reflected by the male nudes that studded his canvases and notebooks, erotic proof of the mystical attraction men have had for each other since Adam fled the Garden of Eden to a land east of Eden known as Nod, where his sons Cain and Abel inaugurated the eternal spiral of murder. The boy Leonardo and his friends were accused of sodomizing was an apprentice goldsmith, Jacopo Salterelli, age 17, a notorious rent-boy. At that time in Florence there existed special letterboxes that citizens used to denounce other citizens. It was in this way that Leonardo and his companions had come to the attention of the authorities. There were two enquiries, at a month's distance, neither of which turned up enough evidence for a conviction, a conviction that held the death penalty. But if convicted one usually got off with a fine and a slap on the wrist, so common was the event. Serge Bramly in his marvelous book *Leonardo* concludes: ''The authorities were prepared to turn a blind eye to various sexual misdemeanors--homosexuality, incest, bigamy: fairly common forms of behavior, after all--on the condition that public order was not disturbed and that a minimum of discretion was observed.'' But Leonardo must have suffered nonetheless now that everyone in Florence knew about his indiscretion, including his father.

Leonardo's exposure to boys was literally limitless. In the workshop artists and their models came and went as they discussed artistic issues and gossiped, most of whom were sexually available. And as Leonardo gained in reputation, he was surrounded by a constantly renewed court of extremely beautiful boys and young men, friends and models, many of which adorned his paintings and notebooks: thighs, buttocks and penises from repose to full erection, or, in his words, ''long, thick and heavy'' to ''short, slim and soft,'' writes Leonardo, and he continues: The male member ''has a mind of its own. When we desire to stimulate it, it obstinately refuses, or the opposite. When a man is asleep it is awake, and when he's awake it's asleep. It remains inactive when we want action, and wants action when we forbid it.'' He maintains that ''it'' can at times be dangerous, inundating the world with human beings the world in no way needs, as well as being the entry point for diseases [syphilis having reached Italy in 1495]. On one page of his notebook he noted: ''A woman's desire is opposite to that of a man's. She wants the size of his member to be as large as possible, while he wants the opposite [in the woman's sex], so that neither gets what he's after.''

Vasari wrote that ''there is something supernatural in the accumulation in one person of so much beauty, grace, strength and intelligence as in da Vinci.'' Da Vinci was also said to be preternaturally gentle for the period, kind to rich and poor alike, generous, always in good humor and possessing a sense of humor. Vasari goes on to say, "Leonardo had such a great presence that one only had to see him for all sadness to vanish." As a person he personified what Plato would call the perfect alloy of *virtu*, intelligence and knowledge. Leonardo was born, out-of-wedlock, in 1473 in the Tuscan hill town of Vinci, near the Arno River that flows through Florence. His father was a wealthy legal notary and his mother a peasant. His full name was Lionardo di ser Piero da Vince, meaning Leonardo son of Messer Piero from Vinci. He lived his first five years with his mother, then with his father who married four times, but never Leonardo's mother. He was a bastard but that had few ill effects in Renaissance Florence, although bastards couldn't be notaries, the position of his father which would certainly have become his own had he been born in wedlock--to the loss of the entire world had his destiny been such. He couldn't become a doctor, either, a pursuit he might well have chosen, given his love of science.

At age fourteen he was apprenticed to the painter Andrea di Cione, known to the world as Verrocchio, in whose *Archangel Michel* we see the incredibly beautiful Leonardo. The choice of Verrocchio was fortuitous as his paintings are exquisite, the demonstration that Fortune never ever stopped looking over Leonardo's shoulder. Verrocchio's shop was in Florence, another lucky break as it was then, as today, arguably the most beautiful city in the world. Verrocchio never married, but this was true of half of the male population of Florence for whom freedom to live their lives as they wished was of prime importance. Verrocchio's apprentices included Ghirlandaio, Botticelli and Botticini, whose *Tobias and the Three Archangels* features da Vinci. At age twenty Leonardo's father set him up with his own workshop, but his love for Verrocchio was such that they worked together until Verrocchio's death. Verrocchio was a father figure, perhaps the most important man in the artist's life.

Verrocchio was described by Serge Bramly as "a sort of one-man university of the arts." He knew and taught literally everything with the exception of huge wall murals, the reason for the disastrous destruction of the *Last Supper*. When Verrocchio was only 17 he had struck a boy, age 14, with a stone, killing him. He was jailed but released when it was proven that the incident had been an accident. Verrocchio was nonetheless haunted by what he had done to the very end, especially as he was a good man. Verrocchio's workshop became the artistic center of Florence where one exchanged ideas, models, recipes for paint and varnishes, where philosophy was disputed and gossip swapped. Of special interest was the new Flemish technique for mixing paint with oil instead of water, making for brighter and more long-lasting colors and smoother gradations of tints, discussed in the life of Messina. Songs were sung and music was played, as Verrocchio was an accomplished musician. He was truly a kind of Pericles who created the conditions for geniuses to thrive--much of which was perhaps due to his attempt to compensate for having killed a lad of 14.

Like all boys, Leonardo liked to dress up and nowhere in world history was there a better, more exciting city than Florence under the Medici. The costumes for festivals and carnivals [designed by Verrocchio and company] were magnificent. Boys' trousers so tight they looked painted on, ample shirts that fell from the collar bones to the upper thighs, taken in by a thin belt at the waist, shirts that scarcely covered the piece of cloth over the genitals, held in place by two ribbons. A headband with perhaps a feather adorned the forehead.

Salaì was the gift of God that those of my sexual persuasion could rightly give thanks for each and every day left to us on earth. A saner man than Leonardo would have thrown him out when the boy stole his first lire, or when caught in bed with another of the master's apprentices. But the genius whom we are all acquainted with, the master of every domain that took his interest, revered the boy as his source of inspiration, as the cherished love of his life. Leonardo could see beyond the daily tribulations and petty treasons. Instead, he held firm to the companion with whom he would walk the rocky path of life, right up to the end. That Salaì was beautiful and beautifully built was important, without doubt, but in a land like Italy, with apprentices he had to turn away in droves, he could have found a dozen replacements. But Leonardo knew that in the end one goes ahead alone or one grants the concessions necessary to share the route with another. The alternative is sterile old age, the shipwreck so well described by de Gaulle in his *Memoirs*.

One of the most impressive realities concerning Leonardo's notebooks is that amidst the thousands of pages there is nearly nothing of a personal nature about the master himself. We have his thoughts, observations, calculations, recipes for mixing oils and ground paint, machines of all nature, fortification, anatomical drawings, male genitalia galore, the texts in reverse left-hand writing, much of which is illegible.

The second love of Leonardo's life was Giovanni Francesco Melzi who became his apprentice around 1508. The boy's father was a senator and a captain in Louis XII's army. Unlike Salaì who only partially succeeded as a painter, Giovanni Melzi did some remarkable works. As handsome as Leonardo had been in his youth, Giovanni followed his master to the end, inheriting half of his oeuvre. The Melzi family property was at Vaprio d'Adda, an enormous mansion, nearly a small Versailles, witness to the Melzi wealth. It was he who informed Leonardo's family of his master's death. Then he returned to Vaprio d'Adda with his master's notebooks and several paintings. He wrote a book drawn from Leonardo's observations about painting, which eventually found its way into the Vatican. The historian Vasari contacted Giovanni for help with the book he himself was writing. About Melzi Vasari wrote, "Sir Francesco Melzi, a Milanese gentleman, entered da Vinci's service as a young and extremely good-looking adolescent. He was very dear to his master and today is a noble and handsome old man."

Leonardo went to Milan where he was happy to put himself under the patronage of Ludovico Sforze who paid him extremely well and allowed him all the time he wanted in order to do exactly what Leonardo himself wished to do, and this for 18 years. Then Louis XII invaded Italy and Ludovico lost it all, eventually imprisoned by the French king until his death. Leonardo, now 48, returned to Florence. The Medici had been expulsed and the Republic reestablished. Savonarola had gone up in smoke and a new breed of artist had arisen, led by Michelangelo and later by Raphael. His father was still there, age 74, with his forth wife and eleven children still at home, aged 2 to 24. Leonardo had written him often, always beginning with "Dearly beloved father…" a tender loving son, even if the reality of their closeness was perhaps other. At age 50 he hooked up with Cesare Borgia who appointed him military engineer, a position Bramly says he deeply desired. Cesare was a bastard as was Leonardo, and Bramly goes on to say: "these two bastard children, having created their own lives, respected each other for their intelligence, independence of mind, and scorn for convention. Leonardo must also surely have been susceptible to Cesare's boisterous elegance and superb bearing." All certainly true as Cesare was virility personified. But unlike Leonardo, Cesare, age 27, was the adored son of his father, Pope Alexander VI, who would continue to love him even after Cesare murdered his brother, Juan--the son Alexander cherished even above Cesare. To have the backing and limitless wealth of his father, the pope, was a huge morale booster. Cesare went on a conquering spree and Machiavelli accompanied him (11).

Both Michelangelo and da Vinci had only their love of men in common. The painted nudes of Michelangelo were peaches-and-cream clean, those of da Vinci homoerotic wet dreams [although Michelangelo's statues were, homoerotically speaking, to die for]. The first, da Vinci, had been handsome, the second, Michelangelo, never. Vasari tells us that it was around this time that a boy, 20, living in Urbino, decided to forget everything he had ever learned about art and dedicate himself to copying Leonardo's paintings, paintings that had just come to his attention. The boy had a magnificent name, Raphael.

In Milan the French reserved a wonderful reception for Leonardo who, for Louis XII, was the reincarnation of the Renaissance itself. He started the *Mona Lisa* but the history of the painting is far to complicated to be approached here. It's the Churchillian riddle wrapped in a mystery inside an enigma. We're not sure even who ordered it, let alone who sat for it, although many think it was Salaì himself. [Michelangelo always had men pose for his statues of woman, as well as some portraits.]

While battles for and against Louis XII whirled around him, Leonardo was creating another work whose importance would span a period of 500 years: it was a study of the human body, dissected with perfection and drawn with a detail that takes one's breath away. In his own words (and 200 illustrations) he tells of accompanying an old man in his last hours, how the man complained of no physical pain, only weakness, and how he gently slipped from life into death. To find out the cause Leonardo did an autopsy, discovering that the artery supply to the heart and lower members had withered, describing, for the first time in the history of medicine, arteriosclerosis. Bramly takes over: "One wonders what it felt like to plunge a knife into the thorax of an old man one had been speaking to not long before." Later in his notes Leonardo describes examining a hanged man, his penis engorged, of which he made detailed drawings. Leonardo went on to say that even if one had a love for dissecting, one's stomach might find it disgusting, and one might "be afraid to stay up at night in the company of corpses cut to pieces and lacerated and horrible to behold."

Finally came his encounter with the man with whom he would end his life, François I, age 19, a giant at more than 6 feet, who loved war, placing himself in the front lines, and was an insatiable womanizer. Da Vinci became François' tutor, and their days and nights were filled with discussion, often in the presence of Salaì and Melzi, all three immeasurable comforts to the old man, old beyond his years as we see in his self-portrait. Personally, I have never, ever come across a life as perfect as de Vinci's; never has there been a man as deserving of the name Man.

The last words will be Melzi's, in a letter he sent to Leonardo's surviving brothers: "He was the best of fathers to me and the grief I feel at his death is impossible to express. As long as I have breath I shall feel an eternal sadness, for every day he gave me proof of a passionate and ardent affection. Each of us will mourn the loss of a man such that nature is powerless to create another."

MICHELANGELO
1475 - 1564

Few men had lived a longer, fuller life than Michelangelo, perhaps none had bequeathed as much artistic wealth to humanity as this tortured genius, dead at age 89, with a chisel still in his hand, at work right up to the end. The body was destined for burial in the Basilica of St. Peter's still under construction, but was stolen by Florentines in the midst of the night, destination a city Michelangelo had not visited for 30 years, his nonetheless beloved Florence. Paraded through the streets to his last resting place, word of mouth spread as to who it was, and soon the streets were jammed with crowds. At the Basilica of Santa Croce the coffin was opened for the benefit of the crowd. The body within was intact, clean and totally lifelike a month after his passing, proof to the assembled masses of the artist's sanctity. But he had not had the luck of going to his tomb in company of his lover, as da Vinci did with Salaì and Melzi. The love of Michelangelo's dreams, Tommasso, was absent, and the love of his life, Urbino, had preceded him in death.

Michelangelo was born a Florentine and he died a Florentine, even if his birth had taken place outside of Florence in Caprese, and he had been destined for burial in Rome. His full name was Michelangelo di Lodovico Buonarroti Simoni, his father was Lodovico who was forced to place him in the bustling workshop of the immense painter Ghirlandaio, at age 10. Forced because the lad was headstrong despite, says Ascanio Condivi, a painter and Michelangelo's biographer, Lodovico's "outrageously beating him." Lodovico had destined the boy for more literary quests, beginning with the obligatory study of Latin, a language Michelangelo would always regret not having learned as it separated him from the ranks of the nobility he admired, a regret that burned like a coal until the day he died. But he did make it to Ghirlandaio's, as if directed by the hand of God, as Leonardo had been fortunate in finding Verrocchio. Michelangelo's older brother, Lionardo, didn't fare as well. Destined for commerce, his father placed him with an abacus teacher, obligatory for the times, Raffaello Canacci, who sodomized the boy, age 10, "often and often from behind," he admitted to the court. He was fined 20 florins and a year in prison which was dropped because he confessed his sin. Lionardo entered the orders, became a Dominican friar, and disappeared from history. Lodovico had five sons about whom he said, "None of them would give me the slightest help or even a glass of water."

In the workshop apprentices learned to look after the tools and keep them clean and in working condition, as well as keeping the shop clean and doing the shopping. They became familiar with the materials used in fresco and tempera, and in the preparation of paints, and how to prepare the surfaces over which the assistants and the master would paint. In exchange for their labor they discovered the secrets of their trade. Michelangelo soon became better than Ghirlandaio, which was bad enough, but he bragged about his superiority in frescoes and tempera to the other boys, earning Ghirlandaio's disdain for the boy's arrogance.

Michelangelo learned about Ghirlandaio's workshop thanks to a boy two years older, Francesco Granacci, who would remain his friend until his death. Together they were sent to work for Lorenzo *Il Magnifico* de' Medici who owed a part of his prestige to his position as patron of the arts. At the moment Lorenzo lacked sculptors and Ghirlandaio sent him the two promising boys. Here Condivi recounts the charming story of Lorenzo coming on Michelangelo as he was sculpting a faun. He pointed out to the boy, then 15, that a faun as old as the one he was creating wouldn't have had a mouth of such perfect teeth. Michelangelo is said to have not been able to hold still until Lorenzo had left so he could knock out a tooth, and then he couldn't wait until Lorenzo returned and admired what he had done. Alas for boy and man, Lorenzo, although still young, had but four years left to live. About Lorenzo the great historian Guicciardini wrote, ''No one, not even his enemies, denies that he was a very great and extraordinary genius''(6). Lorenzo provided him and Granacci a room and a place at his excellent and refined table. Yet despite the refinement, Lorenzo's household was run on an extremely informal basis. One was free to come and go as one wished, and to say what one wished, and Lorenzo himself was always available to boys like Michelangelo, whereas visitors of high rank often had to cool their heels for days before being admitted into his presence. A grown man was present, Poliziano, a professor and Latin poet, a founder of humanism. He translated works from the Greek, especially Plutarch and Plato. He was also a rampant lover of boys, and one can only wonder what effect his intelligence and enticing talk had on seducing the young artist, if any. He took an interest in Michelangelo and was said ''to have loved him greatly.'' Francesco Granacci, on the other hand, would have made a perfect first friend for Michelangelo (he is painted in the nude in the painting *The Raising of the Son of Theophilus* by Filippino Lippi). Another boy was also present, Pietro Torrigiano. He too was a sculptor under Lorenzo's patronage, and later he brought the artistic segment of the Renaissance to England where he finished his life. He was also an insufferable bully and when Michelangelo made some disparaging remark concerning his work, he broke the artist's nose, an infliction that greatly diminished Michelangelo's faith in himself, as he felt he was no longer handsome. [Some say he was Michelangelo's boyfriend and the dispute was in reality a quarrel between lovers, as Torrigiano was known for his startling beauty.] Afraid of Lorenzo's reaction, Torrigiano fled to Cesare Borgia who was offering money to enroll new army conscripts, and as Torrigiano needed money and was physically fearless, he joined his troops. Afterwards, as I've said, he went to England where his destiny was fulfilled.

Michelangelo was called to Rome by Cardinal Raffaele Riario due to a statue Michelangelo had carved and then buried, known as the *Sleeping Cupid*. When experts maintained that it was an example of ancient Greek mastery in sculpture, Michelangelo revealed that it was he the creator. The statue had been bought by Raffaele who had amassed the greatest collection of Greek and Roman art in Rome. Upon arrival, at age 21, Raffaele took Michelangelo under his wing, proudly showing him through his immense collection, offering the boy the chance to do all the drawings of the statuary he wished.

He was commissioned to do the *Pietà*, the money from which he put away in banks or under his mattress. His brother Buonarroto found him living in dingy, humid lodgings, dressed like a beggar. Michelangelo would always live in avarice, collecting and hiding money, and at his death a whole chest of gold was said to have been found under his bed, a fraction of what he had horded away. He never slept enough, ate enough, or dressed warmly enough. He made it known to those around him that he was penniless, perhaps to keep them from asking for alms.

David was next, carved from a block of Carrara marble that had been awaiting the genius, in Florence, for 40 years. Since his early teens Michelangelo had dissected bodies, learning the secrets of tissue, muscles, veins, skin and bone, a grisly, horrifying experience in times without the least refrigeration, a task he's said to have enjoyed, certainly in the sense of a stepping stone to what would become, at age 26, his and the world's foremost masterpiece, *David,* that would reign until the end of time as the measure of perfect manhood. A month after he started *David* he requested that a wall be built, allowing him to continue in private. Nearly two years later, it was removed. The problem arose as to where to put it. So great was its immediate impact that a panel of Italy's finest artists and most prominent citizens, 28 in number, including Botticelli, Filippino Lippi, Piero di Cosimo and da Vince himself--perhaps realizing that the statue would become the symbol of Florence itself--were united to decide where to put it. Months of discussion ended in accepting Michelangelo's own request to place it in the Piazza della Signoria. It was pulled there over greased wooden beams. It was positioned on a plinth and its genitals covered with a garland, and there it would remain until eventually placed in the Accademia di Belle Arti in 1873.

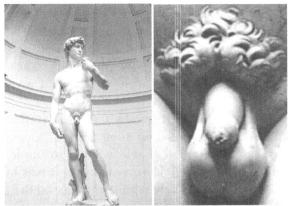

David

The first miracle was its creation, the second is that it has gone through riots, revolutions and wars and has come out unscathed, although nearly immediately four louts were imprisoned for throwing stones at it and had to pay heavy fines. Antonio Forcellino in his wonderful *Michelangelo*, underscores *David's* "provocative nipples ... a penis full of energy ... testicles full of vigor." *David* is the canon of male beauty, now and for always, this gorgeous lad who might have just come out from swimming in the Arno, slightly grimacing at a friend's remark that the water must be cold, judging from his diminished manhood. [More on *David*'s manhood later.]

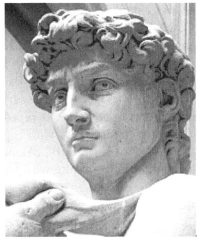

David grimacing

Michelangelo returned to Rome and started work on the Sistine Chapel, painted daily on fresh plaster, a technique of such huge difficulty that even da Vinci is suspected of having given up work on his *Battle of Anghiari* because of his failure in mixing the right components, and then, later, making mistakes when doing *The Last Supper* which, consequently, is lost to us forever. That Michelangelo succeeded on just the mechanics, mechanics on such an incredible scale, is in itself a miracle, not counting, afterwards, the choice of the right oils and right pigments. A patch of plaster to be covered during a day's work was called a *giornata*, the seams of which cannot be seen from afar. Errors could be made up for by painting over the dried plaster, *a secco*. Differences in temperature and humidity complicated the making of the plaster, and the mixing of the colors was a daily challenge, especially as the final result could only be verified once the plaster had dried. Mistakes, when not corrected by painting *a secco*, led to the destruction of the day's work, starting again from scratch. Drawings were made on paper and transferred to the fresh plaster in two ways: In the first the paper, called a cartoon, was held against the plaster and holes were pierced along the lines of the drawing with a sharp instrument; the cartoon was taken away and the holes left an outline of the figures to be painted. Or secondly, the cartoon was pierced before being applied against the wet plaster and coal dust applied over the holes with a cloth. The Sistine paintings are a homage to the male body. In the part dedicated to the story of Noah, called *The Drunkenness of Noah*, Gayford points out that not only was Noah painted in the nude, his sons, shown covering the body while averting their eyes, were also painted--for absolutely no biblical reason--stark naked too. Gayford adds an interesting insight into why the church allowed nudity, saying that it was acceptable because God had made Christ as an incarnation of man, and so the body was not a shameful object. ''Here was a theological reason to decorate the chapel with buttocks, penises, biceps and pectorals,'' says Gayford. The surface Michelangelo had covered was 1,200 square meters, his head looking always upward, compensating with each stroke for the distortions caused by the curved surface. The ceiling was covered with nine biblical scenes, from the division of night and day to the creation of Adam and Eve and the Great Flood. The lunettes, half-moon spaces around the chapel, were covered with biblical ancestors, the pendentives, corner triangles, with prophets and prophetesses. Four years later, at the end of his labors, Michelangelo wrote in a letter to his father, ''I work harder than anyone who has ever lived!'' And it was so.

It is said that in the more difficult portions of the ceiling, the lunettes and the pendentives, he would place a handsome boy, naked, before the area to be painted and shine lamplight from behind him, leaving a shadow on the portion of plaster that he would then outline, a technique that immeasurably shortened the usual preparation. The males served for both men and women.

Sexually, he had his models and assistants, all of whom happened to be among the most beautiful and desirable boys found wherever he decided to set down roots. Michael Rocke tells us of a letter Machiavelli wrote to a friend, describing, in couched terms, what men did at night in Florence, what Michelangelo certainly did: ''A man of my acquaintance went from one site to another that lads are known to frequent, and then wound up finding 'a little thrush' agreeable to being kissed and having 'his tail-feathers ruffled.' After this successful find, the man sealed his conquest,'' as Machiavelli put it, ''by thrusting his *uccello* (dick) into the *carnaiulo* (ass).'' Benevento Cellini writes, in his autobiography, about a youth called Luigi Public ''whose singing was so lovely that Michelangelo, that superb sculptor and painter, used to rush along for the pleasure of hearing him whenever he knew where he was performing.'' The boy became Michelangelo's lover. Cellini goes on to say that Public's father had been beheaded for incest and that the boy had ''just left some bishop or other, and was riddled with the French pox (syphilis)." Cellini nursed him back to health, Martin Gayford tells us, after which the boy had an affair with the nephew of a cardinal and with Cellini's own mistress, in revenge for which Cellini wounded him with a sword. Public was later killed falling from a horse while showing off in front of Cellini's mistress whom the lad was still seducing. Another source tells us that Michelangelo "spent time without end helping boys, like Andrea Quaratesi, to learn how to draw." As Cicero had said of Plato who insisted he was platonic with boys, "If his aim was only to teach philosophy, how was it that he chose only handsome boys and never ugly ones?" The same was true with Michelangelo. Quaratesi was gorgeous, as seen in the master's drawing of him, *Portrait of Andrea Quaratesi*. Cellini tells us that despite the revolts and wars and even the plague, Michelangelo had never seemed more relaxed, and indeed took time to wander around the city, paying special attention to handsome young men.

As Hadrian had found the boy of his life in Antinous, so too Michelangelo found his in Tommaso Cavalieri, who was described as being of incomparable beauty, of having graceful manners, and '"more to be loved the better he is known." Vasari wrote that he was "infinitely more than any other friend" to Michelangelo. Michelangelo sent him a letter in which he said, "I promise that the love I bear you is equal or perhaps greater to that I ever bore any man, nor have I ever valued a friendship more than I do yours." Thanks to Tommaso Michelangelo would know his own Renaissance, a new life at age 60, and he still had 30 years left to share it with this young gentleman. Michelangelo immediately set himself to drawing, the most rapid way to offer presents. One was *Tityus*. Tityus was Zeus' son who tried to rape Leto, in punishment for which he was eternally attacked by a vulture. Michelangelo showed him, in Martin Gaylord's words, being assaulted with "the great bird's groin pushed against his buttocks." [Martin Gaylord is the author of the wonderful *Michelangelo: His Epic Life*, 20015.] Next came the drawing of *Ganymede*, being carried off to Olympus where he would serve as Zeus' servant and bedmate. Then came *The Risen Christ*, a full-frontal nude, followed by *Phaeton*, the son of Apollo who nagged his father until allowed to drive the chariot of the sun. He lost control and Zeus had to kill him before he hit the earth, destroying it. Another highly unique drawing was *The Dream*, showing a naked young man surrounded by a ring of vices, a woman [a man with breasts] awaiting copulation, the exquisite buttocks of another young man, and a fully engorged dick. They were gifts to Tommaso, all accompanied by what would turn out to be dozens of sonnets.

Julius III became pope. He was lucky in that during his reign Queen Mary returned to the English throne and Catholicism was restored, all of which led to his glorification and allowed him to live the lazy, dissolute existence he favored. Added to this was the fact that he possessed great administrative talent and as he had been named governor of Rome twice, he had that center too in his corner. He built an incredibly luxurious palace, the Villa Gioia, adorned by Michelangelo and Vasari and lesser artists who decorated it with Ganymede and other soft-core pornographic satyrs and naked angels.

Like da Vinci and his Salaì, Julius had fulfilled his erotic fantasies thanks to a youngster, Santino, a streetwise urchin of 14 he saw and lusted for. He had his brother adopt the lad who then became his nephew, on whom he showered benefices and named a cardinal, ennobled under the title of Innocenzo Ciocchi Del Monte. He boasted of the boy's prowess in bed, Julius being the bottom to ''his hung boy.''

Of Julius the governor of Milan wrote, ''They say many bad things about this pope, that he is vicious, arrogant and crazy.'' Thomas Beard wrote: ''He makes a cardinal only of those who bugger him.'' The Venetian ambassador to the Vatican, Matteo Dandolo, wrote home to say that ''the pope shared his bed with a boy cardinal''.

After the Julius III's death Innocenzo killed two men who had insulted him in some unrecorded way. The newly elected Pope Pius IV had him arrested and imprisoned for several years, after which he was again arraigned for raping two women. He died in obscurity and was buried, without a funeral, in the Del Monte chapel next to Julius.

Calamity came when Julius was replaced by Paul IV, father of several children, among whom was a merciless killer and sodomite whose savage rape of a young priest cost the boy his life. The murderous son was Pier Luigi Farnese, who would later nearly totally ruin the life of Cellini. He was primitive, cruel, ruthless, decadent, courageous and daring [the perfect subject for a book that, for the moment, doesn't seem to exist], and at age 17 he was already a mercenary soldier in the pay of Venice, along with his brother Ranuccio. Under his father the pope he was given certain lands that he taxed to death, permitting, among his favorites, theft and murder. The boy was so evil that Pope Clement VI had tried to excommunicate him, only to be dissuaded by the bastard-boy's father. Pier Luigi was named head of the papal army, and another brother, Alessandro, a cardinal. Another of Paul's sons, Ottavio, married the illegitimate daughter of Charles V and his boy Orazio married the illegitimate daughter of Henry II of France. Pier Luigi was finally deprived of his miserable existence by Giovanni Anguissola who stabbed him to death and then threw the body, his neck attached to a rope, from the window of Pier Luigi's palace in Piacenza. After all kinds of ups-and-downs the duchy Pier Luigi ruled over finally went to his son [this one legitimate] Ottavio.

Then absolute disaster struck. Francesco d'Amadore, whom he called Urbino, died. He had come into Michelangelo's service as a young man when the master was himself but 30. Michelangelo grew to love Urbino, but in a decidedly different way from Tommaso. Urbino was well cared for, fed and clothed, and he did whatever was needed, from the marketing to the grounding and mixing the paints. But he never received a drawing as did Tommaso. Nor did he merit a sonnet. Yet he was always there. Michelangelo would never put on a clean shirt to greet him, nor, when the sap rose while painting his nudes and he wanted relief, would he need more than pull the ribbons that released the cloth covering his engorged manhood, waiting for Urbino to do the rest. Urbino was always there. Just there. Until he was there no longer. It was then that Michelangelo died, not the biological end that came later. God may not exist but we need Him to exist, He must exist in something, and that something, for Michelangelo, was Tommaso de' Cavalieri. He was the love of Michelangelo's life but not *the* love. That was Urbino, the only person permitted to accompany him during the painting of *The Last Judgment*. Just before the end Cellini had pleaded with Michelangelo to return to Florence, leaving Urbino behind to take care of his master's workshop and belongings. As Cellini related in his autobiography, ''Hearing this, Urbino, in an uncouth way, shouted out 'I will never leave Michelangelo, not until either he or I is under the ground'.''

Surrounded by what the world has to offer in supreme beauty, Michelangelo died alone, having pushed away even Tommaso at the end, thusly sparing himself the cruelest of all destinies, seeing his own ugliness reflected in the eyes of those he had cherished most, the eyes of his lovers, models, assistants, apprentices, boys he met and offered to draw or to teach how to draw, boys in taverns and in allies after dark in a city, Florence, reputed for its warm nights of sublime encounters--with the imperishable boys of imperishable Italy. There would be no Salaì or Melzi at his side. Like Hadrian who lost Antinous, he too would meet his maker alone--the world's supreme artist, not just in his time, but of all time.

CELLINI
1500 - 1571

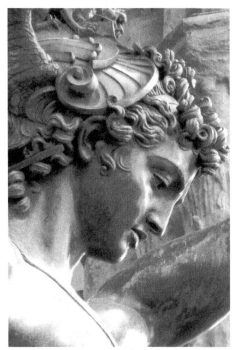

Perseus detail

Giovanni, Cellini's father, was Cellini's first great love, and no son was more adored by his dad than was Benvenuto. He loved the man and the man loved his boy with every fiber of their souls. This was Cellini's first great luck in life. When Cellini went off, they both had tears in their eyes. When he returned, they both wept with joy. In (nearly) the same way, Cellini loved his lovers, boys and men to whom he was fiercely loyal. When Cellini returned to Florence from his first adventures, he came across a former friend who greeted him with kisses and an open bed, and when Cellini went off again, the boy plucked a few nascent whiskers from Cellini's chin to keep in memory.

The second lucky break was being born in Florence. The Florence of that epoch was the most beautiful city in the world, 30,000 Florentines massed between walls that surrounded the town, a space so narrow it could be walked across in an hour. Divided in half by the Arno, where ruddy-cheeked lads swam naked in its refreshing waters, Florence was the birthplace of the Renaissance and home to the hallowed sextet, da Vinci, Michelangelo, Raphael, Botticelli, Cosimo de' Medici and his grandson Lorenzo *Il Magnifico*. Nothing surpassed the beauty of the Piazza della Signoria with its statue of *David*, nor the splendor of the immensely imposing and beautiful Palazzo Vecchio, as well as the Duomo with Brunelleschi's dome, the Baptistery with its Gates of Paradise and the

Pontevecchio Bridge, spanned by jewelry shops that would one day sell, at prices only the wealthiest could afford, Cellini creations.

Cellini's father wanted him to become a musician because all of the great courts of Italy employed them all year round, from festivals to nightly entertainment during dinners. To become a musician was to have assured employment. But when it became clear to Giovanni that his son would never give in, he allowed the boy to join the workshop of Michelangelo Brandini, but took him away after a few months. Cellini may have been removed due to the reputation of artists' workshops, where sex between the master, the apprentices and the models was daily routine. These kinds of relationships were totally par for the course, accepted by parents and society as being the only way boys could learn about life, as girls were shut away. Some workshops, however, gained reputations as nothing more than whorehouses where one could go for sex as one could at any tavern that had rooms.

Florentine sexuality seemed ideal. Men like Cellini passed from boys to girls and back with disconcerting regularity. The reasons are unclear as to why this should have been. Today we're used to a world divided sexually, where there are straights, gays and those who are bi. In Greece women served to keep the home and to produce, basically, sons [although a decree existed that stated that every wife was entitled to sex 3 times a month]. In Rome women were far better educated but were still homebodies, and homosexual encounters were frequent if somewhat smirked at. A Roman woman, unlike Greek women, could really be a helpmate and sincerely loved. In Florence, as we'll see again and again, men--all men--were intimate with boys and other men, despite laws to the contrary, but, again, what is puzzling was the ability to go from one sex to the other with abandon and frequency. Cellini usually took his girls from behind, certainly to avoid pregnancies, perhaps for the increased pleasure of a tighter sheath. Cellini ranted about his boys, covering them with every kind of complement and the most sublime of adjectives: beautiful. He never complimented girls, although about a certain Angelica he did say, in his autobiography, ''I enjoyed such pleasure as I never had before or since.''

By the age of 16 Cellini knew how to protect himself with sword and dagger, as did his younger brother Giovanfrancesco, called Cecchino. ''At that time I had a brother, younger by two years, a youth of extreme boldness and temper.'' In Florence a fight could begin if a boy looked at another a nanosecond too long. For some unknown reason, Cecchino got into a brawl at age 14 and Cellini came to his aid. Several boys were hurt and because boys 13 and over were considered adults, they could have been severely punished. Due to the daily violence in Florence, punishment was harsh in an attempt to keep it down. In the Cellini boys' case, they got off easy, with an order to banish them for a period of six months. They went to

Siena where the goldsmith Castoro, with Giovanni's permission, took them in. Cellini worked on jewelry while Cecchino wandered around the town whiling away time, hooking up with boys and bothering the girls.

It was now 1517 and the seventeen-year-old Cellini had his first real love affair. The boy was Giovanni Francesco Lippi, grandson of the painter Filippo Lippi, and the same age as Cellini. About Giovanni Cellini wrote: "So much love grew up between us that we were never apart, day or night. For two years or thereabouts we lived in intimacy."

A new boy and a new workshop. He entered that of Francesco Salimbene. Here he created a silver belt buckle of supreme beauty, about three inches in diameter, showing leaves, vines and masks. Two years passed and he decided to change workshops again ... and boyfriends. The new lover was Giambattista Tasso, a woodcarver, and one day during a stroll ... but let Cellini take over: "By this time we had reached the San Piero Gattolini gate--the gate by which one leaves Florence to travel towards the Holy City. We looked at each other, tied our aprons around our waists, and set off along the road. It had been God's will that we came to the gates without noticing that we were that far. On the way I asked him, 'Oh, I wonder what our old folks will say this evening?'" Words that ring as true then as today. "I had just reached nineteen, and so had the century."

It could have been the Yellow Brick Road, for it led to a long life of astonishing adventure.

In Rome Cellini and Tasso found work in a shop of Firenzuola. He was well received, especially as he was wearing some of the silver pieces, clasps and a belt buckle that he had made himself. He made a saltcellar that he sold for enough money to wander around the Eternal City and copy the works of art by other artists. He joined a new workshop when his funds were low, that of Paolo Arsago. Firenzuola didn't see things that way and went after Cellini, as he had spent time and money teaching Cellini his trade, but Cellini brushed him off with "As a free man I'll go when and where I please." When Firenzuola lost his temper, Cellini put his hand on the hilt of his sword. "The dispute waxed warm as Firenzuola was a far better swordsman than he was a goldsmith." Luckily a passerby who had been Firenzuola's old master stopped to find out what was going on. He got both talking, and in the end Cellini became godfather to one of Firenzuola's children.

Cellini landed a commission, the crafting of a silver vase, for the Bishop of Salamanca. He spent months on the oeuvre in company of a new lover, this one 14, Paulino for whom, he writes, "I had a passionate love. He was honest and had the most beautiful face I'd ever seen. The love he had for me and mine for him bordered on the unbearable. His splendor was such that he would have driven the Greek gods themselves mad!" Paulino's father met Cellini, and although adventures between men and boys were known and practiced by one and all, there's no indication that he suspected Cellini's attachment to his son. On the other hand, Paulino had a sister that his dad hoped would interest Cellini. "He wanted me as a son-in-law," resumes Cellini in his autobiography. While working on the silver vase he continued his studies in sculpture, drawing and architecture.

As Paulino loved music, Cellini spent many a languorous night playing his flute for the fourteen-year-old who was entranced by his lover's talents, artistry and expertise in the art of virile domination--acquired since Cellini himself was but 13--all of which took Paulino's breath away.

In Florence Alessandro de' Medici, age 19, whose specialty was robbing girls of their virginity, was named ruler of the city by his purported father, none other than Pope Clement VII. To thank the pope and to gain his blessing, Alessandro went to Rome accompanied by a group of boys, louts like him, who came up against even trashier men, the pope's own guard. Among Alessandro's boys was none other than Cecchino, Cellini's brother. The pope's guard arrested one of Alessandro's men--we don't know under what pretense, but Alessandro and his ruffians were known for everything vile, including the mass rape of nuns. The arrested boy, Bertino Aldobrandi, was a friend of Cecchino's--who, like his brother, nurtured extremely intimate friendships with his pals. Cecchino learned, falsely as it turned out, that his friend had been killed by one of the guards. Mad with fury, Cecchino got a description of the man he thought to be the murderer, found him, and "ran him right through the guts," says Cellini. Another guard then shot Cecchino in the leg with a harquebus. The wound festered and Cecchino died. Clement wanted Cellini to return to work despite his mourning, saying that Cecchino was now gone and nothing more could be done. But Italians are extremely bound to their families, and Cellini no less so. He found out who had shot the boy and, as he wrote, "followed him as closely as though he were a girl I was in love with." He attacked him with a dagger, a first blow that grazed the neck as the man, aware of an approaching figure, was able to move slightly out of the way. He tried to run but Cellini was on him like a lion on a fleeing antelope, downing him with another blow, to the back, and as he lay on the ground, another and still another to the neck and upper back. He then ran to Alessandro's palace near the Piazza Navona where guards caught up with him. Alessandro explained the motive for the killing and the guards left. Later, the pope simply asked him if he "had gotten over it now", and gave him a commission.

Cellini got in a row with a jeweler, a certain Capitaneis, with whom he was in competition. Words were exchanged and Cellini scooped up some mud and threw it at him. Cellini *says* that unknown to him there was a stone in the mud and the jeweler was felled. "Provoked by his ugly words, I stooped and took up a lump of mud--for it had rained--and hurled it with a quick and unpremeditated movement at his face. He ducked his head, so that the mud hit him in the middle of the skull. There was a stone in it with several sharp angles, one of which striking him, he fell stunned like a dead man, whereupon all the bystanders, seeing the great quantity of blood, judged that he was really dead." Then a few days later, while sitting with friends outside a shop, Capitaneis happened to pass with some friends. Seeing Cellini, insults and gestures were exchanged. Capitaneis and friends wandered off down the street, giggling. Cellini, despite his own friends who tried to stop him, followed Capitaneis and cold-bloodedly knifed him from behind. Capitaneis' companions had been too surprised to intervene. Cellini is said to have coolly walked away, but when news got to the pope, Cellini's arrest and execution were ordered. Alessandro de' Medici nevertheless gave him a horse for his escape. Later the newly elected pope, Paul III, gave Cellini a pardon and a commission saying, "Men like Cellini, unique to art, are above the law." Cellini nonetheless decided to join Alessandro in Florence.

When Alessandro took power in Florence he said, "They made me duke, so I'll enjoy it!" By enjoying it he meant wandering the streets at night fully armed, pushing aside anyone in his way, looking for a fight he was destined to win for the simple reason that he had barred the carrying of a sword or a firearm, both of which never left him, nor did his dagger. And he had reason to fear, as the nobility of Florence wanted him replaced by legitimate blood, noble blood. He had gained power at age 19 and had by now fully tasted every perversion, so that what was left was taking the hymen of those who still had one, notably nuns, and that of those who kept guard over theirs, virtuous women. He liked his boys too, for quick, easy couplings, as heated and virile as possible. His favorite companion was his cousin Lorenzino with whom he shared his bed and more when not extinguished from a night of whoring. And when he awoke with a lustful urge, Lorenzino was always conveniently spread out, naked, at his side. This is how Cellini had caught them many times, as the artist was permitted to come and go as he wished, and as Alessandro had no modesty and no need to hide his vices, Cellini was aware of every thing that went on. "Meanwhile I went on making the Duke's portrait and oftentimes I found him napping after dinner with that Lorenzino of his."

No one knows why Lorenzino turned against Duke Alessandro, aided by a professional assassin, Scoronconcolo. In his play, *Lorenzaccio*, Musset writes that Lorenzo wanted the duke dead so that Florence could become a Republic again. Others suggest that he was just jealous of the duke's powers and privileges. As Duke Alessandro was so unpopular, he was never without his body armor, weapons and guards. But Lorenzino told him that he had found a Florentine lady of exceptional beauty and, especially, ironclad virtue, who had been abandoned by her husband. Lorenzino would bring her to the duke, and from then on it was up to the duke to prove that he could triumph over virtue. Lorenzino convinced the duke to dismiss the guards for the night, to take off his armor and to slip naked into bed. From then on it was easy for Lorenzino to strike him with a dagger. Afterwards he rode off to Venice, a glove covering a finger Alessandro had nearly bitten off. There, he published his version of what had taken place in his *Apologia*, claiming to be a second Brutus. Lorenzino himself was later stabbed to death by a poisoned dagger on a bridge in Venice.

Cellini decided to exchange Italy for the court of François I , a king who had been trying to allure Cellini to Paris for years. What happened between them can be found in the chapter on François. After he returned to Florence.

There he went to find Cosimo I de' Medici who had replaced Alessandro de' Medici. Cosimo had not been taken seriously as a young man, his priority being himself and the quantities of drink and women his young body could do honor to. So all were surprised when he not only took control of the government, but also had his enemies tortured and beheaded in public. Pleasure and pleasurable surroundings were in the de' Medici blood, and that which was true of all the rich--a need for art in the form of paintings, frescoes, sculptures, drapery, sublime clothing, silverware, magnificent gardens and fountains--was true on an even grander scale for the de' Medici. Cosimo promised that if Cellini produced a great work of art, he would not be disappointed in his reward. Cellini suggested doing the statue of Perseus, Cosimo agreed, and thus began the countdown to Cellini's Immortality. The year was 1545.

A place for it was rapidly found, in front of Cosimo's home, the Palazzo della Signoria, facing Michelangelo's *David*. A new boy, handsome, naturally, was found too, a very young lad, Cencio, son of a prostitute who would eventually accuse him of sodomizing her boy in an attempt to extract money, but for the moment that was in the future. He took on Bernardino Mannellini, the exquisite head and body of whom would be the model for the future *Perseus*. ''He was 18 and I asked him if he would enter my service. He agreed on the spot. He groomed my horse, gardened, and soon essayed to help me in the workshop, with such success that by degrees he learned the art quite nicely. I never had a better assistant than he proved.''

If you've read my book *TROY* you know that I'm mad about Greek mythology. But frankly, the story of Perseus isn't all that passionate: Acrisius, King of Argos, wanted a son and consulted the Delphic Oracle who told him that his *daughter* would have a boy, but that the boy would grow up and kill Acrisius. So Acrisius locked away his daughter, who was nonetheless impregnated by Zeus who took the form of a golden shower (?). The son she bore was Perseus. Acrisius refused to kill them both so instead locked them in a chest that he flung into the sea. The chest was netted by fishermen loyal to King Polydectes who reared Perseus. Polydectes wanted to marry Perseus' mother but Perseus refused him her hand, telling the king he would give him whatever else he wanted. The king said he would settle for the Gorgon Medusa, a monster having a terrible face and hair of serpents, a face so horrible that the person looking on it froze with fright. The gods favored Perseus and gave him a sack in which to put the head, winged feet to get to it, a sickle to cut it off, and the helmet of invisibility belonging to Hades. Perseus collected the head and returned [after profuse adventures] to Polydectes who said he had sent the boy away to be killed by the Medusa, and had never planned to give up his mother. Perseus opened the sack, looked the other way, and froze Polydectes to stone. He then returned to Argos where, during Olympic-style games, he threw a discus that rebounded and killed Acrisius.

In 1548 Cellini cast the figure of Medusa and in 1549 work on the rest of the statue began. It was around this time that he hired another handsome youth, Ferrando di Giovanni da Montepulciao, who would cause him much grievance later one. Just before the actual casting he fell sick with fever, brought on, certainly, by the incredible stress related to his work. Luckily Bernardino Mannellini was there to see that things went along correctly.

Perseus comes through as a real living youth, his brow knitted as is Michelangelo's *David*, his look grave. The body of the Medusa is just as living, just as wondrously human.

A marble block had been brought to the workshop in 1549 to serve as a base for *Perseus* and in 1552 Cellini cast two figures which would go into the block, Mercury modeled after Cencio and Danaë modeled by a new girl Dorotea. When Cosimo's wife saw the two figures she wanted them for her own rooms but not only did Cellini refuse, he also sealed the figures into the marble base with such firmness that they could not be removed. Cencio, as *Mercury*, is totally naked and eminently desirable. He had shared Cellini's bed since the age of 12. Dorotea also shared his bed and gave him a son he legitimized. She also accommodated Cencio. All told, Cellini was living and creating, creating and living, in the most beautiful city in the world, under skies warmed by the unstinting generosity of Helios, his *Perseus* complete, his Immortality guaranteed.

The last years of his life seem to have been marked by increasingly ill health and unattainable projects. From Paris the immensely original Catherine de' Medici requested that he return to his Parisian palace to build a tomb for her beloved husband, Henry II and for herself, two kneeling figures. Health and insufficient willpower prevented him, but he was tempted. He was part of a committee that arranged the burial of Michelangelo whose reputation--in death at least--now placed him, in the eyes of mere mortals, among the gods. He made some trinkets, jewelry, seals and buckles as he had as a very young man. He left his fortune to the de' Medici, asking only that they care for the boys in his workshop.

He went to work on his book which, next to *Perseus*, was his greatest triumph. He was aided by a boy, age 14, and seemed to have liked the experience of talking about himself while the lad noted all.

He weakened. He died, accompanied to his resting place by hoards of admirers--I can't say *last* resting place because, for this man who had never stopped moving, it was, in reality, his first. When I entered the Peace Corps, a very young boy, I received a huge box of books, as do all volunteers. One was *The Autobiography of Benvenuto Cellini*. I read it with great pleasure, totally unaware of the volcano who had produced it, only vaguely aware of my own sexuality, never dreaming that I would eventually, like countless other boys, fall in love with this incredible creature, proof that God truly does work in entirely mysterious ways (1 and 13).

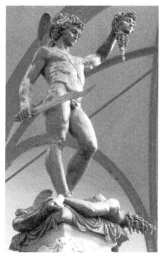

Perseus

VINCENZO DANTI
1530 – 1576

Born in Perugia, Danti is another sculptor we know little about. He received a commission for a bronze statue of Pope Julius III whom we met in the life of Michelangelo. Like many workers in bronze, he was influenced by Donatello, whose effeminate bronzes do not enter into a book dedicated to the virility of the male phallus. He took part in a contest with Cellini for the construction of the Fountain of Neptune [although Bartolomeo Ammannati won], which brought him to the attention of Sforza Almeni who commissioned *Honor Triumphs Over Falsehood* represented here, a magnificent work carved from a single block of marble [although nothing is comparable to the above *David*].

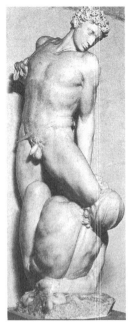

Honor Triumphs Over Falsehood

And finally, just for the hell of it, I'll end with the big-dick artist himself, Beardsley.

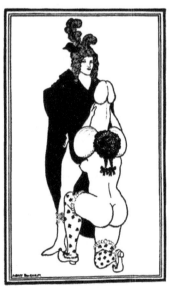

Lysistrata: Adoration of the Penis.

18-year-old Beardsley (Aubrey, 1872-1898) was retained by Oscar Wilde to illustrate his works, especially Wilde's *Salomé* when Beardsley was 20, and Beardsley was one of the few to remain faithful to the playwright to the end of his life. Beardsley was known for his Art-Nouveau illustrations in black ink. He had traveled to Paris where the influences of Toulouse-Lautrec and the Parisian passion for Japanese prints changed the artistic direction of his life. He stated that his own ambition was the grotesque. He dressed as a Wilde-like dandy, and sexually could have been anything from asexual to insistent rumors that he impregnated his sister. He converted to Roman Catholicism as did Wilde, and requested that his obscene drawings be destroyed--they weren't. Suffering from tuberculosis, he withdrew to Menton in France (my own second hometown), as had Le Gallienne, where he died at age 25.

MALE NARCISSISM

In our times the symbol of masculinity is Parris Island and the Marine Corps, yet a whole subculture has grown up concerning Corpsmen whom we see on the Net in the throes of every imaginable kind of homosexual sex. It's strange how nearly all marines resemble each other, displayed in footage of marine locker rooms and showers. The same stocky builds--slim, narrow-waisted marines seem not to exist--the same haircuts and USMC tattoos, down to the exact replicas of their genitals. Entirely naked, they give each other close-crop haircuts and unselfconsciously spread out in the sauna, displaying full pubic bushes. Others openly shave their bushes while taking a shower, at times brushing their teeth under the spray, and openly pissing. One Marine wrote a wonderful book about his gas station in Hollywood where he supplied fellow Marines and girls to actors. The writer, Scotty Bowers, was in his 90s when he wrote *Full Service*, and his Marines liked the men they serviced because they were rich and had swimming pools and took very good care of them (9). In *Some Like it Hot* Jack Lemmon tells Tony Curtis that he's going to marry Osgood. Why would a guy marry a guy? asks Curtis. Lemmon's answer: *For security!* In European showers men are completely different from Marines: tight pectorals and flat bellies, dicks of all lengths, all uncut, some with balls in tight scrotums, while others hang incredibly low, and their asses are mostly hairless and firm. For Italians the word modesty is nonexistent, and that from ancient times, and one who is well hung will, today, gladly exhibit himself in a locker room or pull it out for curiosity seekers who have heard of a certain boy's dimensions, if asked nicely and if the supplicant is supposedly heterosexual.

[Speaking of pissing: Pissing standing up, in Marine showers or elsewhere, is one of life's pleasures, so when German women protested that it was unhygienic when done in toilets [because men's poor aim occasionally wet the seats], and demanded that men sit down, like women, I was shocked to read that apparently 40% of German males kowtowed!]

A man's manhood must not be questioned, as he will kill to prove it, shaking off every intellectual warning to not do so. In war, in duels, men gladly go to their deaths as long as they'll be remembered as having been men in life. Being accused of a lack of virility is a man's worst humiliation, and one he will avenge or, if killed, have avenged for him. A case in point is Richelieu's beloved father: Armand Richelieu's father François was chased from his family when, as a boy, he murdered a local noble because the noble had had François Richelieu's brother assassinated over a seating dispute in the local church. François Richelieu's mother, a redoubtable Nemeses, kept the coals of revenge burning in François Richelieu's heart until he was old enough to kill the noble, a plan that consisted of his waiting in a nearby swamp that the man had to cross. When the man's horse entered the muddy banks François cast a cartwheel at its legs, obliging it to rise up, casting the noble into the water where François ran to plunge a sword into his chest. The authorities ordered his body broken but François escaped to Poland where he became one of Henry III's mignons--sexually or not is unknown, but probable. He then returned to Paris with Henry who was crowned king at the death of his brother Charles IX. François Richelieu had been one of Charles's pages before killing the noble, his brother's murderer. François went on to father two daughters and three sons, one of which would become the great Richelieu, Armand Richelieu. (10)

We may have seen the peak of masculinity a generation ago, the one that fought the last world war. They may have been shorter, but a picture of boys and men then show them all wiry and lanky, all with superb pectorals and narrow waists, all smiling contentedly despite the dire conditions, surely because they were happy to be together, but also because the American Dream was more and more at their fingertips. The same boys today are obese or getting there, are smirking binge drinkers and have or will one day have stupid tattoos and ridiculous piercings, they'll belong to rifle clubs and swallow righteous religious gobbledygook. They'll naturally believe in God and Mom, but the first will not have the slightest say over their daily lives, and the second will have less influence still. In a word, *all that for that.* [Tut-tut.]

A European boy will take the time to prepare himself a well-balanced meal in the tradition of his parents and their parents--he doesn't need guidance from health magazines. Of course, Americanization will eventually win out because Europeans are less and less able to pick and chose among American values as shown on t.v. and in films, more and more inclined to fast food and fast fixes. Being a man today often involves fast driving and chalking up the highest numbers of hits on girls [of dubious value due to today's inexhaustible and willing supply]. Death-defying sports are a must because the quality of life has fallen to the extent that one hardly cares if he dies. When I arrived in France a boy was lucky if he had his first car around age 30 or more. Today, like in America, it's offered by his father [offered by enlightened fathers if their sons will forego the certainty of physical injury or death by not buying motorcycles].

It's more and more difficult to distinguish, today, between egotism and narcissism. The normal definition of a narcissist is someone who can't sustain satisfying relationships, has difficulty with empathy, is hypersensitive to insults or imagined insults, is vulnerable to shame, loves flattery, detests those who don't admire him, uses other people like disposable Kleenex, and often exaggerates his achievements.

Freud believed there was a healthy narcissism necessary in personality development, but after reading several texts on the subject it's obvious to me that not everyone agrees just where healthy narcissism ends and pathological narcissism begins. Freud wrote that pathological narcissism was simply an extreme manifestation of healthy narcissism. Certain psychologists differ over whether narcissism is healthy or not, whether it's even a disorder, and even whether it's a defensive or an offensive response to a situation.

Most of us certainly work on cultivating a self that exudes authority, control, knowledge, competence and respectability. It's the narcissist in us all, a way of not appearing stupid or incompetent.

Men are narcissists and sex provides the narcissist with everything vital to his existence: power, self-esteem, the whole supplemented by the excitement of the hunt, the thrill of attracting someone using nothing more than his beauty and charm--at the same time reinforcing his confidence in both. Homosexuals like to add the element of danger [docks, parks, toilets], an adjunct that hugely stimulates the libido and assuages boredom, the whole capped with an erect penis and the boy on his knees feeding on it, the wonderful pressure building in the balls, and a body-shaking orgasm, the expulsion of streams of semen, visible proof of his manhood. Most of the men in this book, from Alcibiades to Laurence Olivier, were the charming and seductive, the intelligent and worldly, proof of this.

All men are narcissists, but what is called bad narcissism can be recognized in an infallible way: he will always be friends with someone until the person no longer serves his purpose, after which he will find a reason for severing ties between them, one that *always* leaves the narcissist blameless for the separation that the other person somehow deserved. He takes what he wants, and moves on. Because of his need to protect his ego, he offsets criticism with anger, or he retreats, the other left to face the punishment inherent in his withdrawal. There is little or no give-and-take, very limited flexibility. Moving on from one person to another is only doing what every man would do, were he not hampered by societal or religious handcuffs, believe these narcissists.

And perhaps they're right. Perhaps millions of years of evolution-- billions if one counts back to the first amebas--have made men the way we are in the unique aim of perpetuating the species, the bee whose destiny *is* to fly from flower to flower, immortalized in Rogers and Hammerstein's *The King and I*, so that his seed will be distributed over the greatest area, between the thighs of the greatest number.

Many narcissists have high energy levels and favor any physical activity that will enhance the beauty of his body, especially, today, weight lifting, and the ever-crucial beauty of his face [although yesteryear limp-wristed Etonians wouldn't have been caught dead anywhere near a gym (8)].

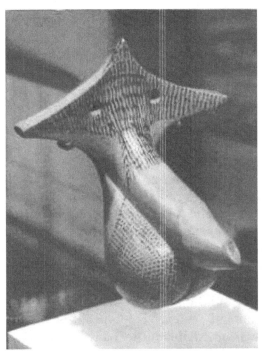

The phallus, an object of supreme beauty: A terracotta vase dating back 2500 years, used to store perfumed oils.

Many homosexual narcissists claim to have had deeply emotional experiences with women, even if psychologists maintain that they are misogynists who not only hold women in contempt, but go so far as to loath and fear them. Strange when one considers the love, often excessive, they had for their mothers, an exclusive relationship that many of the same psychologists believe is the very root of their homosexuality. Psychologists divide homosexual narcissists into two categories, somatic narcissists that I've described above, and cerebral narcissists who often prefer masturbation to sex with a real person--W.H. Auden an example (8), who often isolate themselves socially--the original Garbo ''I want to be alone''-- and, like Garbo, most often *do* end up alone. What is of importance to them are intellectual pursuits, sports and politics, and they're capable of forgoing sex for long periods, although, add psychologists, during ''life crises'' these men often turn to intensive sexual activity as a way of lessening stress. The crippling of one's image of self, the wreckage directly due to aging, leads to depression and, depending on how much his image of himself is based on his physical impact on others, can end, in the absence of an alternative road, in self destruction.

Just as we have not advanced beyond the Kinsey Report with new studies, so too are we blocked, as in a time machine that refuses to advance, in the theories of Freud, who divided a boy's sexuality into three zones, and three periods, each lasting a year and a half. Today these exact same zones remain, our major erogenous zones.

The first is the mouth, through which kissing will procure immediate and extremely deep emotional and sexual fulfillment, in some ways more satisfying than directly touching a boy's member, and includes nursing a lad's nipples prior to descending and embracing his sex, pleasures initiated through the mouth just moments after our birth, at the breasts of our mothers. Freud claimed that those of us frustrated during this stage, those who couldn't have milk on demand, as it were, led to personalities characterized by pessimism and envy, while those who had an abundance became optimistic and generous towards others [and are, often, gullible].

The anus as an erogenous zone can be of such import that boys and men crave penetration, although others fear a simple thermometer. Reaming is little practiced by heterosexuals, but homosexuals, whether they want to be penetrated or not, know that it is one of the most sublime moments in male-male sexual love. It is also an erogenous zone for infants, and although we can't remember that time, Freud maintains that parents who let their children do as they wished during toilet training, making no demands, produced adults who are messy, careless and disorganized. Strict parents, or parents the child does not wish to please, going when *he* wishes to go, produce what Freud called anal-retentive adults, someone neat, precise, stingy, withholding and passive-aggressive.

The phallic phase is the most vital of the three. Here the boy's sexual desire is concentrated on the penis and involves his natural love for his mother, a love he feels is blocked by his father who is in the way. The boy becomes aggressive towards his father-rival. When the boy sees that he cannot have his mother because his father does, he identifies with him, becomes as much like him as he can, so that he too will one day have a female of his own. If, on the other hand, he feels he cannot win the battle against his father, and thereby identifies with the passivity of his mother, he will want what she wants, a male for her bed. This is the root of the boy's homosexual fixations, the catalyst of his narcissism. In other forms of sublimated rebellion against the father the boy turns to self-expression through art, or he may turn to crime, the reasons boys who choose these alternatives can so easily swing between heterosexual and homosexual activity, which both artists and prison inmates are open to.

It's impossible to define narcissism better than the definition found in *Wikipedia*, that I'm going to quote: ''The key to understanding narcissism lies in the myth its name comes from: Narcissus falls in love with an image, a reflection of himself. While the common understanding of narcissism is being in love with oneself, the reality of narcissism is being in love with an *idealized image of oneself.* It is believed that deep down, narcissism is self-hatred, which results in a rejection of the real self, or 'true self', and the fabrication of a 'false self'. The narcissist is therefore someone who, like Narcissus, has lost himself in an illusion.'' [My emphasis.]

In a sense, all boys are in love with themselves--their egos, needs and wants coming first. But a healthy narcissist is one who accepts and loves himself, while another category of narcissist rejects his true self.

The root causes of narcissism are not only disputed, but appear contradictory. A boy can be treated as being so special that he deems himself above others. When the reality around him shows that he is not, he turns to illusion. Or the opposite, he is treated in a way so shabby that he becomes ashamed of who he is, and thusly chooses a new self to mask the former shameful one. A child who is punished for what he does may evolve into a ''good'' boy who skirts his parents' conception of what is bad by putting up a false front, one that contents them while burying his true self. Or the child may have felt abandoned or neglected during infancy, and lessens the impact of his suffering by creating a new self that is non-emotional, and while other boys learn from trial and error, he clings to the unemotional person of his creation, his growth irredeemably stunted. The hustler Denham Fouts, portrayed in my book *American Homosexual Giants*, lived his whole life as if he were a teenager, and could only have fulfilling sex *with* a teenager. Even in appearance, boys who are loved and boys who are not are as different as a black hole from the sun, the lustful spark of life absent from their eyes.

Narcissists live for themselves, an immense deliverance from the societal obligation of marriage and producing a family, freeing them to lead their lives in exactly their own way. Because no law binds them to their occasional friends, they can cut themselves free when the other is no longer of value. Narcissists are unforgiving and vengeful, and a frequent arm used by narcissists is the silent retreatment, or they sulk. They abandon the person while playing on what is their own deepest fear, being themselves abandoned, or they abandon the person first, to protect themselves from being abandoned later. And it was perhaps this, the primordial fear of abandonment, that made them narcissistic in the first place, an incident or series of incidents during their childhood that they've forgotten or deeply buried, but which drove them to create an inner world with its own stability, and once they had created that inner being, they would never ever abandon it, so terrible had been the chaos and lack of structure during their first years.

They never forget an affront and dream up plan after plan on not only how to get even, but how to come out ahead. They are extremely sensitive to criticism, and were they writers, one bad review would wipe out a thousand good.

Expressions commonly used for narcissists are "emotional vampires" and "emotional black holes". There's no limit to whom a narcissist will eliminate if a person is no longer needed or has become a weight; being a family member, a brother or a sister, is no guarantee of a narcissist's loyalty. If a narcissist feels threatened he will unleash hell. Any dent in his armor becomes life threatening. Nothing is too small to escape his attention and feed his fear. He sees things in black and white, and basically has just two gears, kind forbearance or, when opposed, boundless rage. Any threat to his control will trigger immediate intimidation, that will advance to plots of revenge and physical abuse. Thousands of married narcissists have chosen the expediency of murder to rid themselves of spouses, uncaring of the destruction wreaked on their children. Luckily for homosexuals, they're free to simply walk out the door [although porn star Chris Lance's life ended in murder (4)].

THE IMMENSELY BEAUTIFUL PHALLUS

Lance and Novotný

Because of their physical perfection and incredibly huge and beautiful phallus, two men represent the paramount in phallus worship: Lance [David Allen Reis] and Pavel Novotný [Jaroslav Jirik, aka Max Orlaff and Jan Dvorak]. Their lives and full naked frontals, their members hard and soft, can be found on Amazon in my book *Hustlers*.

Lance
[David Allen Reis]
1962 - 1991

Lance and Leo Ford were a perfect on-film couple, and in real-life they paired to hustle together, as trade was instant pocket change, and L.A. clients often filthy rich. Lance packed 9" of the thickest uncut beauty in porn history. Blue-eyed and blond, he was 5' 11" and weighed in at 160 lbs. His life is an enigma, an incredible shame because he appears to have been intelligent as well as gorgeous. He is thought to have lived in foster homes and he went to Capuchino High School in San Bruno, California. He lived on and off in San Francisco and purportedly had a thing for Latin boys.

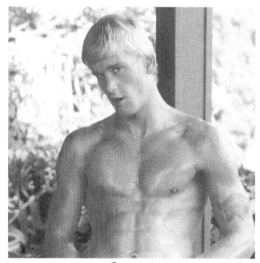

Lance

Porn star and hugely talented porn producer and director William Higgins (4) talked about his preference for heterosexual Slavic boys, boys who work very hard for very little money, unlike professionals like Novotný who performed only when he chose the partner he wanted, and then he did it his way. Of course, good chemistry is a means of assuring a good scene, and as I've personally never seen a creature as physically perfect as Novotný, perfect in face, body, muscularity and a cock whose size and beauty defies imagination, I suppose he deserves a certain amount of latitude. Those who possess the rights to his films are guaranteed a fortune, it seems to me, until someone better comes along, which is hard to image. For me the beauty of Novotný is timeless, and his face can only be compared with the perfection of the famous sculpture of Nefertiti.

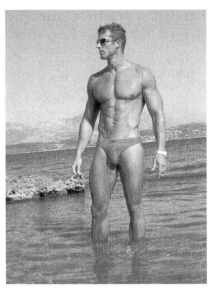

Pavel Novotný, aka Max Orlaff and Jan Dvorak, born in 1977 in Prague, Czech Republic. 6' 2''. Pavel is a BelAmi boy, boys well-endowed, who don't shave their pubic bushes [although they are trimmed], physically *crème de la crème*.

I would like to end this chapter with a glimpse into the life of a boy every gay boy dreams of meeting, Mike Henson.

Kenneth Walsh wrote an excellent book, *Wasn't Tomorrow Wonderful? A Memoir*, 2014, on growing up in a perfect family, finding out he's gay, first sex and first boyfriend, to his winding up sharing an apartment with two guys, one of whom turned out to be Mike Henson, and their night together that followed. Ken's book is intelligent, well-written, amusing, the true step-by-step of a boy going through boyhood into gay manhood. The book is the proof--from this thoroughly clean, honest boy--that no matter how much you love, no matter how much you want to be faithful and loyal, the attraction of the next boy, and what's hidden beneath the buttons of his jeans, the curiosity, the discovery, the mystical worship of the phallus, new lips to kiss, new nipples to caress, will win out every time. You end up doing what Mike Henson and his live-in boyfriend did, you throw a pool party and pass a night of bliss with the new guy on the block.

After ending his career in porn, Mike began working in computers, doing programming and software maintenance. He graduated from the UCLA School of Computer Sciences. David Forest, a producer who made *Seed Money: the Chuck Holmes Story*, wrote: ''His [Mike's] performances were some of the finest ever filmed. He was one of the most versatile, sexy, 'real' male stars that ever worked in our industry. AND ... in real life ... he was just the sweetest, nicest, happy-to-lucky, 'boy-next-door' you've ever met.''

Mike lived with an army buddy and boyfriend, Dennis, who found him dead on returning home, from a drug overdose, a Bible in his hand.

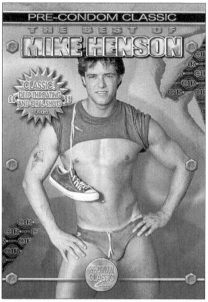

Mike Henson, one of the sweetest boys who ever lived.

Male beauty includes pubic hair that crowns the phallus and adds to the visual impact of the male genitalia. It's strange that heterosexual males have adopted the homosexual fashion of shaving the pubic bush, just as they blindly adopted, for a while, purses for men.

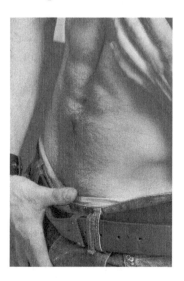

Pubic hair took years to grow and represents what is most masculine in men. The boy above reveals just enough to get the onlooker, male and female, eager to see the rest.

SIZE AND LIES

We won't spend much space on the size of African members, because they're simply *hors-catagorie*, a little like comparing an Ethiopian sprinter with your garden-variety occasional runner. The Hebrews claim that the Curse of Ham was the origin of African penile immoderation. Ham was cursed either because he didn't cover his father, Noah's, nakedness when he came upon him sleeping, or because he copulated aboard the Ark. The curse was his blackness and monstrous appendage, a curse used during colonial times to justify slavery, blacks being considered as inferior [because cursed]. Christianity had indeed stooped low, and even President Jefferson, himself a slaver, said, concerning slavery: "I tremble for my country when I reflect that God is just."

The prolific writer James Cleugh stated that under the pharaohs Ethiopians were hired to deflower wives because the Egyptians had a fear of vaginal blood. Ethiopians had been gladiators in Rome and caught the attention of those curious about their manhood, as they were at least as often nude as dressed. Today's Egyptians often have enormous phalluses, the heftiest among Arabs. In 1774 Edward Long wrote his *History of Jamaica* and noted the extravagance of male protuberances, something I can testify to because I lived on the island for two years, and something of deep interest to English girls who had plantations there or worked on the island, as in this example taken from my autobiography (1):

Had I been on less intimate terms with Jamaica I might have feared that I would be spending a part of my time protecting the volunteer from crazed white-flesh hunting rapists. But in the Jamaican countryside, crime was little known, and rape unnecessary. Whites were as protected a species as the koala bear. Once Johnny, a superbly handsome charcoal Jamaican, called in to see me after a visit to the factory doctor, a fiftyish Bristol matron.

"My sex was hurtin' me," Johnny said.

"What did she say?"

"Keep out of Greenhouse Hotel," he snickered.

"How did she examine you?"

"She make it hard."

"Hard!"

"She always make me get it hard when I'm hurtin'."

"What does she do?" I asked.

"She feels to see where it hurt."

"Christ! Has any other white woman ever touched you?"

"The plan'er's daughter. She see me when I bring a package to her mamma. She say coma ah here, Johnny. She say let me see it."

"Did you?"

He shook his head, grinning from ear to ear. His expression reflected the folly of a black messing around with a white girl. The thought was there; but buried in a hundred years of subjugation.

And this written about an excursion to Bath:

Up the Main Road was Bath, a village of flowers and thermal springs where a volunteer from Linda's group, Mary, was stationed. Mary was proud of and entirely devoted to the Jamaican family with whom she shared her three-room shack. For all purposes a nun, Mary took nourishment--like bacteria-feeding nodules--from the haven of an ideal.

"I'm a virgin, you know," she announced to me at the Cascades one day, making Linda pull a long, how-does-she-dare-come-out-with-things-like-that face and turn away blushing. I was left gaping, not so much at the confession as at the incredible solemnity of the declaration, as if she'd admitted to having a venereal illness.

Me too, he could have by rights answered, and added that it was little indeed to blow one's horn about.

Mary was kind and generous, very short in stature and still on the decent side of chubby. She had wiry black hair and wore a huge crucifix between two mounds of mesmerizing amplitude.

From the village of Bath we hiked up a trail through luxuriant jungle to the Cascades, a dozen basins of water as clear and ice-cold as the glaciers of the Tetons. We sunbathed on the marble-smooth banks and dove in when our skin became flushed. Occasionally we came upon bathing blacks and mixed-blood East-Indians, like Buba. Their naked virility squelched any thought I ever had of going nude, and I could only pity Linda's future husband whom she would appraise along these outlandish standards. Unlike Sophie, the volunteer from Louisiana who unhesitatingly used the word dick, Linda and Mary neither saw nor spoke evil, but an increase in their lighthearted chatter betrayed a repressed anxiety. Although I admitted to myself that I went to the Cascades in the hope of such encounters, I felt guilty that Linda thought I rode all those kilometers just to be with her.

The English explorer Richard Burton (2) measured African dicks as part of his research for his *magnum opus*, *The Scented Garden*, 1,282 pages long and was *said to have been* a defense of homosexual activity, a work his wife read and destroyed after his death [and she had him buried religiously, something Burton had specifically requested *not* to take place].

Where Burton found African members to be 6" long when *soft*, French surgeon Jacobus Sutor found the Sudanese possessors of 12" cannons. He wrote *L'Amour aux colonies* in 1898. He was stationed in Asia, Africa, South America and the Pacific islands, and was said to have used his position as a doctor and an imperialistic white man to measure every dick that came his way, and there had been hundreds.

David Friedman in his excellent *A Mind of Its Own* brings us a comment by a soldier, William Feltman, who in 1781 was invited to a dinner at an American table, the servers black slave boys who wore only shirts. "I am surprised this does not hurt the feelings of the fair Sex to see those young boys of Fourteen and Fifteen years old to Attend them, their whole nakedness Expos'd and I can Assure you It would Surprize a person to see those damned black boys how well they are hung."

The Egyptians collected the phalluses of their enemies, as did an African tribe discovered by Vasco da Gama, about which a traveler wrote: "When they kill any of their Enemies, they cut off their Privy-Members, and having dried them, give them their Wives to wear about their Neck, of which they are not a little Proud: For they who have the most are most esteemed, in regard that Evidences the Husband to be the more hardy and valiant. It was as great an honor as it is with us to wear the gold Fleece, or the Garter of England." A quote brought to us by Nigel Cliff from his *The Last Crusade, The Epic Voyages of Vasco da Gama*, 2011.

There's no dispute about Nature's generosity to the inhabitants of the African continent, but there is great dispute concerning size elsewhere.

The problem is that institutes which bring us information concerning penises at rest and aroused depend on the measurements made by the men themselves [although Kinsey personally went to incredible hands-on length in his research into male sexuality, his own sex life was rich and enriched by the students he had access to, one of whom was Gore Vidal (much more on Kinsey later)]. In Kinsey's 1948 *Sexual Behavior in the Human Male*, after receiving the penile measurements of 3,500 men, he came up with an average 6.2", ranging from 4.8" to 8.7". The shortest was 1", the longest 10.5". [Tom Hickman states that in his classes Kinsey loved to ask girls to name the human organ capable of the greatest expansion. The girls would at first blush and then look foolish when he gave the answer, the iris of the eye.]

Masters and Johnson called the penis "the great equalizer" because penises that looked extremely short when soft could outgrow penises that looked, soft, very long, once they erected. There supposedly no correlation between flaccid and erect dicks, which I personally find hard to believe.

As I mentioned in the section on Greek and Roman sexuality, small penises were found esthetic for the first, and for the second those well-endowed were applauded in the baths. For the first, the Greeks, big members were considered ugly, course and the tools of barbarians, whereas in Tel Aviv, Hickman tells us, a poster campaign to humiliate bad drivers said, ''Research proves aggressive drivers have small penises.''

The perfect boy, for Aristophanes [in *The Clouds*], had ''a gleaming chest, bright skin, broad shoulders, tiny tongue, strong buttocks and a little dick.''

Men check out other men, it's a fact, and in a survey for *Playboy* 2/3rds of the men wanted ''something more in their shorts'', and in *The Hite Report on Male Sexuality* the majority of the 7,000 men interviewed ''wished they were bigger''. To get there, weights, pumps and stretching devises are used, even a simple elastic band connecting the glans to a band around the thigh, worn under one's clothes. The Arab technique of *jelq* is popularized on the Net, and involves stroking the erect phallus from the base to the tip, over and over and over again, the commentator giving the man the choice between ejaculating at the end of the exercise or saving himself for release with a companion [see *ErosErotica*--the lad magnificently hung and the film highly erotic]. Men are undergoing operations to increase both length and thickness, with the same ardor as women who want breast implants.

Kinsey
1 man in 100 reaches 8''
7 men in 1,000 are beyond 8''
1 man in 1,000 reaches 9''

Durex Studies
5.5 men out of 100 reach 8''
35 men out of 1,000 reach 9''
20 men out of 1,000 go beyond 9''

The Durex average of 6.4'' is extremely close to Kinsey's 6.2'', and if we combine both we get an average of 6.25''. [From a Durex Global Sex Survey, 2005.]

These measurements were *all* self-measurements, whereas in a large 2001 Lifestyle Condoms survey of 400 men who did *not* measure themselves, the average came out 5.8'' [14.928 cm.], a *huge* difference from Durex and Kinsey. [During the Lifestyles Condoms measurements each man was measured twice by two nurses working in tents, ''protected by gloves''. Of the 400 men measured, only 75% could get a measurable erection. [LifeStyles Condoms is an Australian company, previously known as Pacific Dunlop Limited.]

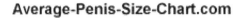

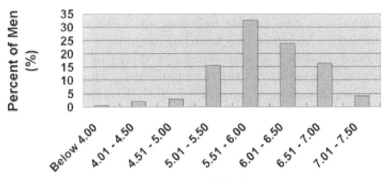

It seems natural that a guy with a 5 ¾'' rod will allow himself 6'' when filling in a research report. Researchers believe that men who think they're small will shun studies where someone is going to measure them hands-on, as in the Lifestyle Condoms studies, researchers who will then perhaps giggle behind their backs. So they won't take part, which means that the hands-on average of 5.8'' may in reality signify that the average man is smaller still.

As the vast majority of a woman's pleasure comes from the area directly outside the vagina, and the first two inches within, a man's penis, states Jared Diamond, Pulitzer-Prize-winning scientist, is therefore several times bigger than biologically necessary.

All men take their size very seriously, but gay men much more seriously than others, that I personally can testify to. And when I see the dick sizes of the boys in BelAmi porno I want to know who did the operations, for how much, and at what time is the next plane to his office [more elsewhere concerning enlargement techniques and the lives of history's super studs].

Grigori Potemkin's power over Catherine the Great was said to reside in his instrument that he would show one and all when he strode through the Winter Palace naked under his unbuttoned dressing gown. Errol Flynn left the door of his dressing trailer open, and showed himself in full erection, an invitation to any boy or girl wishing to relieve him. Truman Capote was bedded by Flynn, an incident that would have been rapidly forgotten had it not been the famous Errol Flynn, wrote Capote, which suggests that he had found Flynn small. About the Kennedy brothers, who loved to skinny dip, Capote said all three of their rods would have to be added to make one of normal size. In a club, when a man whipped out his for Capote to sign, Capote said, ''Well, maybe I can *initial* it,'' a similar response to Oliver Reed's equipment which he hauled out at any moment, in bars and even on a plane, one woman yawning, ''Is that it?'' The priapic Grigori Rasputin proved to a doubting crowd in a restaurant that he was indeed the man who had infinite influence over the tsar and tsarina by exhibiting himself. The crowd had heard of Rasputin's reputation for being hugely endowed, and was now no longer in doubt of the man's identity. Later, Rasputin's assassins cut off the instrument, which reappeared in a Saint Petersburg museum of erotica in 2004, looking like an over-ripe banana a foot long, Tom Hickman tells us. His manhood had measured 33 cm/13 inches.

Milton Berle ''was world class'' and artist Eric Gill drew his constantly.

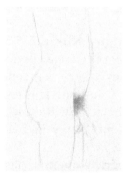

Gill Self-portrait.

Alpinist George Mallory had himself photographed nearly exclusively in the nude (2).

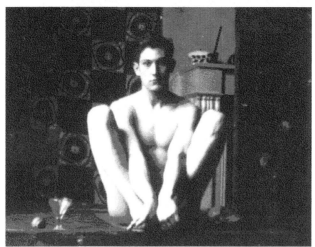

A photo of Mallory taken by Duncan Grant. Mallory asked Grant for copies of the photos he took, stating, ''I am profoundly interested in the nude me.''

Tarzan Johnny Weissmuller put his to use at the Garden of Allah swimming pool, showing and demonstrating it in action during the wee hours of the morning (3).

Alfred Kinsey biographer James H. Jones wrote, concerning Kinsey, ''he seldom passed up an opportunity to show off his genitals and demonstrate his masturbatory techniques to staff member.'' He ''had very large genitalia, and that means both penis and balls.''

In Robert Caro's magnificent books on LBJ, Johnson would go naked in front of his school friends, saying, ''Wonder who we'll fuck tonight?'' while seizing his purportedly huge dick.

Rank	Country	CM	IN
1	Congo (Braz.)	17.93	7.06
2	Ecuador	17.77	7.00
3	Congo (Zaire)	17.33	6.82
4	Ghana	17.31	6.81
5	Colombia	17.03	6.70
6	Venezuela	17.03	6.70
7	Lebanon	16.82	6.62
8	Cameroon	16.67	6.56
9	Iceland	16.51	6.50
10	Sudan	16.47	6.48
11	Jamaica	16.30	6.42
12	Panama	16.27	6.41
13	Nicaragua	16.26	6.40
14	Benin	16.20	6.38
15	Brazil	16.10	6.34
16	Peru	16.03	6.31
17	Puerto Rico	16.01	6.30
18	Haiti	16.01	6.30
19	Georgia	16.00	6.30
20	Dominican Republic	15.99	6.30
21	Burkina Faso	15.89	6.26
22	Czech Republic	15.89	6.26
23	Denmark	15.89	6.26
24	Senegal	15.89	6.26
25	Gambia	15.88	6.25
26	Netherlands	15.87	6.25
27	Belgium	15.85	6.24
28	Zambia	15.78	6.21
29	Belize	15.75	6.20
30	Italy	15.74	6.20
31	Angola	15.73	6.19
32	Egypt	15.69	6.18
33	Zimbabwe	15.68	6.17
34	Bosnia	15.67	6.17
35	Hungary	15.61	6.15
36	Paraguay	15.53	6.11
37	Nigeria	15.50	6.10

Phallus size per country. The Czech Republic is 22nd, while judging from Czech porn, it should easily be first.

Being hung is in itself lucky, but the bigger the dick the longer the foreskin, foreskins that not only cover the glans, but can exceed it by a good inch. Guys with big balls produce more ejaculate, a win-win-win for those that have all three, a long shaft, a long foreskin and nice-sized testicles.

In *La Nuit de Noces* by Al-Suyuti we read: ''When a man's instrument rose to its full dimensions she exploded with joy, and welcomed it. It must be said that a good virile instrument is 12 inches in length, or 3 times a closed fist; while others are 6 inches, or a closed fist and a half. Some men have 8 inches, or 2 times a closed fist. Women have nothing to expect from a length of 6 inches during copulation.''

The size of the phallus is of ultimate importance in Arab stories. In Mohammed Cheikh Nefzaoui's *The Perfumed Garden* we have the story of the wife of the great vizier who wished to possess the clothes of the court jester. He said that he would give them to her in exchange for a night of coitus. When the wife hesitated, the jester recounted a series of lecherous tales, which put her in an erotic mood. The jester took advantage of the moment by revealing his member, a huge pillar that she seized and examined, astonished by the size and beauty and rigidity.

In another story one women tells another, her neighbor, how satisfied she is with her husband, who has an immense shaft that stretches her vulva to its limits and penetrates her full length. The instrument possessed by the neighbor's husband is too small to give pleasure, the reason for her unhappiness. That night the neighbor perfumes herself and enters the couple's bedroom and bed, on his side. Awoken, he immediately stiffens at the smell of the perfume and enters what he thinks is his wife, but is surprised at the narrowness of the sheath not used to so large a weapon, and also at touching bottom before being completely inserted. After they've both spent, he withdraws and she returns to her bed. The next morning the husband, disoriented by a night of strange perfumes, imagined that it had all been an erotic dream.

THE GLORIFICATION OF THE PHALLUS THROUGH CLOTHING

No Greek boy would have imagined today's trends in designer underwear because the boys then were as naked, under their robes and chitons, as modern men in kilts.

Romans wore the subtly-named subligaculum:

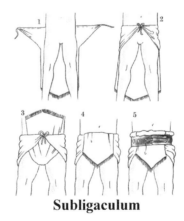

Subligaculum

From Codpiece to Jocks

The moment of glory for boys and boys' wear was the Renaissance, as we see in this extract from my book *Cesare Borgia*:

Cesare addressed Juan as his Lord brother, and admonished him to give thanks to their father, Pope Alexander Vi, who had made the family so great. Juan was married in Barcelona to a young cousin of King Ferdinand and Queen Isabella. Given everything he could wish for from birth, Juan spent his time whoring--and his young body was capable of giving him a great deal of pleasure--drinking and gambling. It's not known if he ''honored'' his wife on their wedding night, so decided was he to go off with his friends to shatter the quiet of the Barcelona night. Juan was clearly Alexander's favorite, another supposed reason for Cesare's hatred. As virile as his father, slim waisted and certain of his sex appeal, Juan swaggered through the streets of Rome in what can only be described as gorgeous attire, a cloak of gold brocade, jewel-encrusted waistcoats and silk shirts, skin-tight trousers with drop fronts--cloth attached by ribbons that would free a man's loins when he wished to piss and fuck. This beautiful, gorgeously clad body, stabbed nine times, 30 golden ducats still in his belt purse, was fished up from the Tiber, to the grief-stricken horror of his father who locked himself away from public view for three days. The death freed the way for Cesare to renounce his vows, having been made cardinal at age 18. Alexander VI never confronted his son with the murder of his favorite boy, but that he was guilty was silently acknowledged by nearly all. On the morning of the murder, just before sunrise, men were seen leading a horse with a body strapped over its back to the river edge, untie and then caste it into the middle. They were accompanied by another man on a white charger, his silver stirrups and gold spurs reflecting the moon's glow. The men, said the witness, a Slovenian watchman standing guard over boats carrying cargo, spoke in very low voices … in Spanish.

The cloth that covered the genitalia made access rapid and the bulge signaled what the boy had to offer.

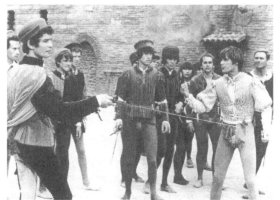
Renaissance manhood on display.

Unlike American and French boys, Italian lads are always toying with their flies, touching, stroking, gently caressing the covering fabric, a rite they share when they're together, an erotic exercise that girls pretend not to notice. Italian boys are the only ones in the world who can wear yellow, green and even red trousers and come off looking perfectly virile. Their ease with their bodies is astonishing, and they seem to not hesitate to show themselves before their mothers and sisters in briefs, even in the morning when they are tumescent, or slightly so.

During parts of the Middle Ages and the Renaissance codpieces were in fashion, emphasizing the male groin, growing in size and volume as the years passed, and one man tried to outdo another. Worn to boast, they kept a man decoratively contained.

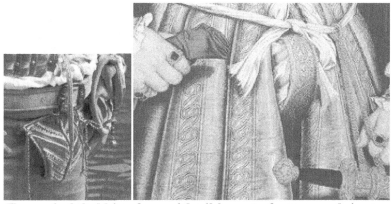

From cloth held in place with ribbons to fortress codpieces.

Codpieces were even found in suits of armor. It was probably a mode, although some suggest that it originated to hide bandages around syphilitic penises, and it's true that codpieces were popular in the 1500s, during the worst of the syphilis epidemics [purportedly brought to Europe with the return of Christopher Columbus]. Cod was Middle English for scrotum and in some places it is apparently still used as a term for the male genitalia.

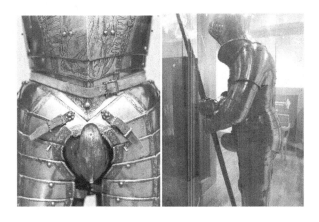

The codpiece was also a kind of genital shield, protecting a guy from being kicked in the balls, or his dick being otherwise harmed, and during the Second World War soldiers in airplanes sat on their helmets, preferring to protect their lower head rather than the upper. Dicks have always been an endangered species: the Egyptians collected them as trophies in the thousands, as did Emperor Hadrian in Jerusalem, castrating living Jews, asking them how they could consider themselves the ''chosen people'' when already mutilated through circumcision? For hundreds of years, during the Middle Ages and the Renaissance, men were put to death by having their genitals cut off before being disemboweled and quartered (6), and during the Protestant Reformation thousands of lads were emasculated by Catholics, the ultimate insult (5). During the French Revolution of 1789 the penises of decapitated aristocrats were shown to the crowds, and during the Protestant massacres under Henri III the genitalia of Protestant men were cut off and shoved in their mouths, forced open by their assailants.

Footwear grew along with codpieces because phallus size has *always* been equated with foot size. The shoes were called poulaines and at first tapered off at 6''. But like codpieces, they soon were extended, some to 30'' and had to be held in place by strings [or silver chains] attached to the knees. Edward IV finally had their length limited to 24'' for nobles and 6'' for commoners.

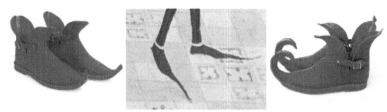

Poulaines

Money pouches became fashionable, called a *bougette* from the French *bouger*--to move. Attached to the side or the front, the swinging pouches, when allied with a dagger, boosted a male's morale and were suggestive to females of those other, hidden attributes.

Da Vinci wrote that men should not be ashamed of mentioning and displaying their manhood, advice Elizabethans turned their backs on with the advent of puff shorts, in the center of which one could just barely make out a tiny codpiece, fitting for the court of the Virgin Queen.

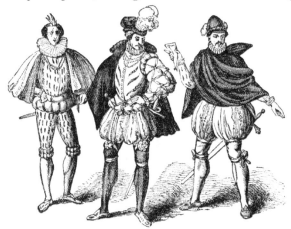

Puffy shorts and codpiece now nearly invisible.

Like girls who have to pretend they don't notice Italian boys perpetually toying with their toys, so does one have to pretend nothing special is being exhibited during today's ballets that flaunt packed baskets. Matadors lead "with more than their chin," writes Hickman, with leg tissue stretched over what appears to be huge male organs. [A young matador was filmed dressing, his equipment encased in a kind of gauze that held it in place before he tugged on his suit of lights--maddingly erotic.]

In the early 1900s workers in America wore union suits, often of red flannel with buttoned front and buttoned-up flap in the rear. It was replaced by W.W. II long johns in two pieces, of huge importance in winter conditions, thermal and still worn today as never-bettered wear to keep warm, the jogging suit and other sweats the more fashionable alternative.

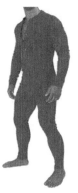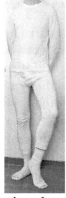

One-piece red union suit, two-piece long johns.

Boxers and briefs share the field today, the first allowing the beast room to roam, the second snuggly protective and wondrous for showing off one's equipment. The combination of jeans and briefs has never done more to promote male beauty, second only to the Renaissance, the reason I've chosen a Renaissance image for the cover of this book.

During the 1970s boys wore trousers cut high into the groin, disclosing their potential, a mode that accentuated, at the same time, their small marble-hard buttocks. And basketball shorts were the right length:

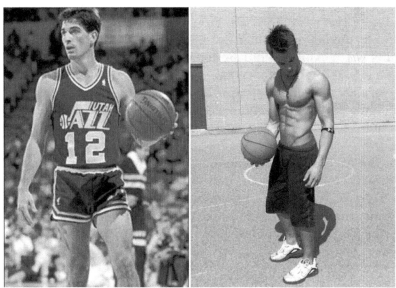

Shorts then, shorts today. Imagine the boy on the right without all the excess tissue.

After the extinction of the codpiece men found ways to accentuate their groins by the use of anything from handkerchiefs to bunched-up socks, and in the film *Hair Spray* one lad was obliged to remove dough-roller-sized padding he'd tucked down his crotch.

Homosexual models differ from heterosexual models in that homosexuals *always* wear designer briefs, some cut to emphasize a boy's pride:

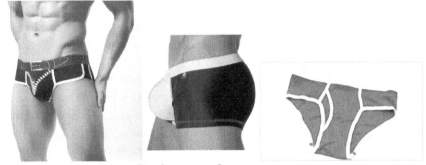

Designer underwear.

Hickman informs us that men wearing kilts were obliged to be naked underneath, and they were checked with mirrors attacked to the end of sticks into the 1960s to make certain that this was the case.

In this extract from my book *American Homosexual Giants* we see the incredible evolution in American mores, this example dated 1949: ''Bill Harris, for a short time with Isherwood, was Jack Fontan's longtime lover. Jack, an actor, was in the cast of *South Pacific*. Director Joshua Logan, seeing his physique, had him strip off his t-shirt and with a pair of scissors Logan cut away Jack's shorts, his balls apparent when he stretched out over the sand in the theatrical version of the play. When women in the front rows complained, Jack took to wearing jockey briefs. Logan found out and was furious, 'If they don't want to see his balls, they can have their money returned.' ''

Ewan McGregor was apparently not unhappy to expose himself nude in *Velvet Goldmine* [with what looks like an entirely normal 6''] and Kevin Costner, nude in so many of his films that I know his dick nearly as well as I know my own, said he would sue if a certain shot of him nude was cut from the film. Rob Lowe showed an ass to die for in *Youngblood*, and then filmed himself screwing a gal alongside a buddy, Lowe's fully erect dick seemingly normal in size but no less an erotic wonder [visible on the Net].

We'll end with what goes under the shorts, back then as well as today:

I was accompanied by my mother on my very first rendezvous with a jockstrap, in the sports department of Salt Lake's very chic Arbachs (pronounced Arbahz by the moneyed and Arbacks by the hicks). The gentleman wanted to know what she wanted, and *she* seemed determined not to tell him. Sign language followed and all I remember is wanting to hide under a carpet. What happened next has been mercifully erased from my memory, although I did leave the store equipped for gym and the world of men that awaited me.

I never found jocks particularly sexy until I saw Rob Lowe in *Youngblood*, as stated, where he paraded in front of a girl in a jock and then turned around and walked away, inciting an admiration for Rob that hasn't left me to this very day.

Originally developed for cyclists and delivery boys on bikes, they were invented by the Bike Company in 1874 and the company has held its first position ever since, offering jocks today in a blue that would make Yves Klein red with envy. They were obligatory in my school days but apparently not now. I personally find that briefs offered as much support, but the argument seems to be that the uncovered ass permits better evaporation of sweat. For violent sports like karate a plastic cup in the jock is a must.

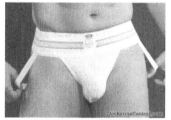
Jockstrap

MALE ENHANCEMENT

Phallus enhancement differs markedly from breast enhancement in that the latter is relatively safe, the former still considered dicey. Men want to look big in the locker room, but it's an arms race. If one guy enlarges his dick the others will want theirs to be bigger still, with the risk of losing, forever, the great hard-on one's born with [literally: boys are born with erections or get them immediately, one doctor stating that he had to race to cut the umbilical cord before boys erected]. A bigger dick will increase self-confidence in some, and make horsing around with pals in the showers and towel snapping more fun. [Men often die with erections too: Tutankhamen's embalmed penis stood at an angle of 90-degrees.]

Boys always compare themselves with other boys, the reason they want their dicks to look long when flaccid, although the comparison usually goes much farther, as in circle jerks destined to see who can cum the fastest, shoot the farthest and with the greatest quantity of ejaculate, and who's hung and by how much.

Girls don't appear to get all that hot and bothered about big dicks, their preference being active tongues and forceful fingers powered by powerful biceps. 85% judge their partners' phallus size satisfactory against 55% of men who "felt good" about their own equipment. Men are truly from Mars, women from Venus. Women need love made to the whole body while men need something warm, tight and humid. Studies claim that 20% of women never have orgasms, that half fake it, that only 25% have orgasms regularly, while women have incredible *latent* power, capable of having orgasm after orgasm after orgasm, "skimming like a stone across water," states Hickman, perfectly. [Masters and Johnson claim that a woman with a vibrator can have 50 consecutive orgasms.] The clitoris has twice as many nerve endings as the penis, and is "virtually inexhaustible ... the only human organ purely for pleasure," concludes Hickman. [After doing quite a bit of research, I can assure the reader that the results of certain statistics, like the frequency of female orgasms, can vary *immensely*.]

Of course, men have orgasms, boys one after another with but little pause, their peak reached between the ages of 15 and 17 [already over-the-hill at age 18]. The question of who, the woman or the man, has the most pleasure in sex was resolved in ancient times by Teiresias, as disclosed in this extract from my book *TROY*. Zeus and Hera, as usual, are arguing:

"I can no longer put up with your continual complaints," flared Zeus. "All I want is a warm hearth with steaming ambrosia and a stout nectar; my pipe filled, my socks darned, and my favorite chair cleared of dogs. I ask no more than the most common of mortals. I know of mere peasants who live in greater comfort than I.

"But look what I provide you in return. I give you palaces, slaves, rule over the gods, a daily change of robes and sandals, dominions in Heaven and on Earth, plus islands, your own herds and flocks, rivers and lakes, not to speak of countless subjects and a personal Oracle. As for that snide little comment about our bed, don't forget that our honeymoon alone on Samos lasted three hundred years. Each fortnight you're honored with my presence, and since the pleasures of the boudoir are far greater for women than for men, you enjoy much more satisfaction that I--my flirtations included."

"You're insane. Everyone knows that a man has more pleasure in love than a woman."

"Nonsense. The opposite is true. The proof is that men talk a great deal upon the subject when among themselves to compensate for the lack of the real thing. Whereas women--harlots excluded--keep quiet about it because they are satiated and because if men knew about the enjoyable time women have, they would all want to change their sex. Who would be left then to provide you with your play toys?"

"That's the most outrageous, the sickest thing I've ever heard. But wait. Would you like to put what you've said to a test?" challenged Hera.

"Here you go scheming again. Can't you remain one minute without hatching some new plot?"

"This is no plot and anyway it's you who've asked for it," began defiant Hera. "Listen: One day the mortal seer Teiresias came upon two serpents that were coupling and killed one of them, the female. As always happens in such cases, Teiresias was turned into a woman and spent seven years as such until one day she came upon two other serpents coupling and killed the male, becoming herself a man. He has therefore lived the life of a woman and a man and can tell us who is the receiver of the most pleasure. Would you agree to calling him?"

"I would indeed," accepted Great Father. "Apollo! Apollo!" From the orchard appeared a splendid youth.

"Yes, Father," said tender Apollo in dutiful compliance.

"Go to earth and bring back Teiresias," ordered Zeus.

"That's not necessary, Father," said the young lad. "He's here himself. Athena has turned him into a woman for spying on her in her bath, and he's come to ask you to change him back."

"Ye gods! *You* do it, and then bring him here," commanded quick-tempered Zeus.

"As you see, Husband, if it were so pleasurable to be a woman, why would Teiresias want to be turned back into a man?" concluded self-satisfied Hera.

"That we'll find out right now. Here he comes."

Teiresias, an old man with long, faded hair and an effeminate gait shuffled in. He wore a tattered, purple robe which trained on the floor as he came forward.

"Come here, Teiresias. My wife and I would be grateful if you could shed some light on a rather age-old problem: During ... uh ... the act of love, who has the most pleasure, the man or the woman?"

Hera and Zeus anxiously awaited the answer that was unforthcoming.

"Well, good man, don't leave us in the dark," prodded Zeus.

"Tell my husband what he wishes to know," urged Hera, leaning towards Teiresias, whose quivering lips were on the verge of parting.

"What am I to say?" began frightened Teiresias, looking from the goddess's stern, sagging jowls to Eternal Father's craggy, once-handsome face. "Which of you am I to obey? I'm sure that if I answer that it is men who have the most pleasure, I will receive blows from one of you; while if I answer that it is women, I shall be set upon by the other."

"Have no fear, dear fellow," assured humane Father. "I give you my word that I shall not harm you, and you know that the word of a man if his bond."

"I'm certain one of you will become angry and take revenge upon me," sniffed Teiresias.

"Speak. No one will hurt you," cooed Hera, fingers crossed.

"If I knew which of you was for what..." essayed Teiresias.

"No!" shouted Hera, knowing that Zeus' power would ensure him the vote. "We want only the truth!"

"Would you repeat the question?" quaked Teiresias.

"Of course..." started Zeus.

"It's my turn!" interrupted Hera. "The question is: Who has the most pleasure during sex..."

"Mother!" cried puritanical Father.

"...the *man* or the woman?"

"So as not to offend either of your godlinesses, let me answer with a little verse that you can interpret as you wish."

"Oh, the coward," fumed Hera.

"He's been a woman too long," concluded Zeus. "But say your verse. If it's too obscure we'll take it to one of the Oracles."

"And it'll come back a dozen times less intelligible," said Hera. "But proceed. Tell us your little poem."

Timidly Teiresias began. "If the parts of sexual pleasure he counted as ten, thrice three go to women, only one to men."

"Ha, ha, ha," rejoiced Zeus.

"You mischievous scoundrel," raged Hera, and in her furious anger she blinded Teiresias by casting a baneful spell over him. She then stormed out of the room.

For homosexuals bigger is always better, a need fired by pornography in which guys are chosen for their dick size, and in Slavic countries like the Czech Republic heteros try out for gay films more often even than gay Slaves, which brings them vast sums of money [in comparison to what they earn in factories], so the competition between the boys is cutthroat, where only the cutest, the enormously hung, win out. To this is added enhancement techniques that studios like BelAmi have the secret to. When your everyday gay lad sees these huge dicks he judges himself super small, and so penis enhancement becomes *the* only solution. Even back in Al Parker's time Al made lots of extra cash by going from sex shop to sex shop selling penis pumps, exiting with his pockets stuffed with dollars for the orders placed. He himself used the pumps before filming scenes, so he knew he was selling something that worked (4). [Although pumps have apparently no long-term effects.]

Where surgeons once refused to operate on a guy who had 4'' or more, today a whole new industry has developed, entire clinics dedicated to giving a patient exactly what he'll pay for.

90% of all penises measure 3 to 5'' soft, 5 to 7'' hard. The blood pressure in the phallus is twice that of the body in general, and it takes 2 ounces of blood to fully charge the beast. The purpose of the following is to make certain both take place:

Surgery

Surgical enlargement of the penis can aid in gaining 3 to 4 cm [1.18 inches to 1.57 inches], the visual impact more noticeable flaccid, exactly what a guy wants in order to impress his buddies in the showers. Most men believe that deeper penetration will give a greater orgasms to a woman, but as a woman's nerve endings are on the outside surface and innerly to a depth of 2'', this is not the case.

An incision is made in the pubis area at the place where the penis is attached to the body, and the suspensory ligament is severed:

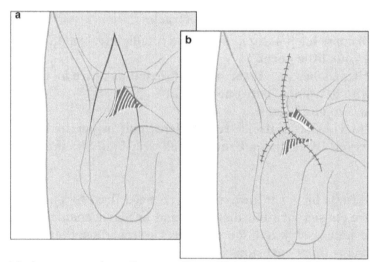

(a) shows area where the operation will take place, (b) is post operative, showing the cut ligament and skin realignment.

The operation allows the penis to move farther forward. It is normally performed in a hospital for easy access to pain medication and erection-blocking drugs. A guy is back to work in a week and back in the saddle in a month.

The risks are loss of erection angle, erectile dysfunction, nerve damage and documented deaths. Clearly stated, the risks associated with surgery far outweigh the benefits. Also, weights or stretching devises are necessary after surgery to insure that the penis does not snap back into its original position, perhaps even *becoming shorter than before.*

The surgery costs $15,000, adds an inch and cuts the ligament that makes the erection erect, meaning it no longer salutes as it used to, and you may have to put it, manually, into whatever erotic opening you favor.

Two urological researchers, Marco Ordera and Paolo Gontero of the University of Turin, examined 230 men, half who had undergone surgery and half nonsurgical procedures. They found that those who had had surgery had a high rate of complications. Those who used traction methods [to be discussed] resulted in growth of around 0.70'' [1.8 cm] when flaccid and 0.67'' [1.7 cm] when erect. In all cases the traction method had been used from 4 to 6 hours daily, over 4 to 6 months, those who went the full 6 months showing slightly longer rewards.

Girth can be obtained by wrapping strips of AlloDerm [recycled human tissue] around the rod or down the shaft. 1-2 cm [0.40 to 0.78''] can be gained which, in girth, is noticeable. The dick head can also be augmented through injections under local anesthetic; the procedure takes an hour and lasts a year. Specialists in California offer triple penile augmentation, length, width and head in one operation. As usual in Hollywood, there are plenty of guys who vow they're now sporting 2 extra inches in length thanks to surgery, and one soldier acknowledged the respectful looks he now received in the showers, which seems to have been his aim. But *all* publicity concerning surgery is suspect.

World-wide, Germans go in for phallic enhancement surgery more often than other nationalities, perhaps because Germans are so well endowed that those who aren't feel ashamed, and so correct it by surgery. In Brazil the men are enormously endowed, but surgery for Brazilians has become such an accepted way of life that it is often a case of big not being big enough, a phenomenon fond in Brazilian women's breast implants, often of staggering dimensions. The U.S. is in the 4th place, but this is certainly temporary as more and more centers are opening, especially in California, dedicated exclusively to penis enlargement.

Traction / Extenders
[Also called Tugging]

This involves 6 hours of traction daily for 6 months, the end result adding from 1.8 to 2.3 cm [around an inch--0.70 to 0.90] at rest, 1.7 cm hard [0.66''].

The extender places the penis under tension, creating micro-tears in the cells which, when repaired, make the penis longer. They can be worn under the clothing.

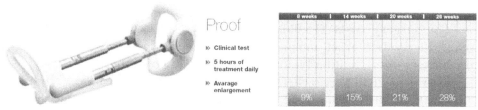

The device and the statistics furnished by the constructor of the device.

Extenders do not increase girth, which women find more pleasure-giving than length.

One source indicated that traction could possibly harm the glans and its nerve endings. The penile head is a membrane similar to that of the inner eyelids and lips, but remarkably thinner; it is not your usual skin. The glans was an internal membrane until robbed of its protective covering through circumcision.

The bottom line is that traction is easy to use, it seems to give results as least as good as surgery but without the incredible risks of surgery.

Gentle milking through jelqing is a pleasant adjunct.

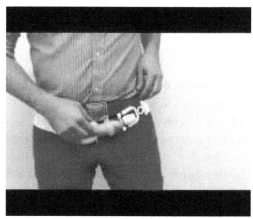

Worn under the clothing.

Pumps

Pumps are cylinder devices that fit over the penis and create a vacuum. Blood rushes into the penis, engorging it. Pumps provide temporary size enhancement, and are otherwise universally judged as ineffective.

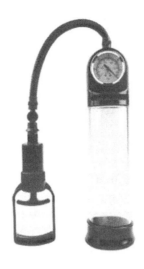

Jelqing

Jelqing is practiced 30 minutes each day for months to enlarge the penile cavities, whose that fill with blood, making for longer and larger erections [although, as usual, some doctors warn about nerve damage].

Form an OK-grip around the base of the phallus.

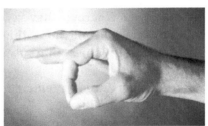

OK-grip

With light pressure, slowly move your grip up the well-oiled shaft of the penis, stopping just before the glans. It should be done while the phallus is 50 to 100% stiff. Each repetition takes from 2-3 seconds, and after each you alternate hands. There is micro-tearing, that will increase both length and girth as it heals. For the first month use only a medium pressure grip in order to develop penis strength and resistance. Jelqing is also an exercise in self-control, not immediately cuming, restraint that will come in handy when you're in your partner.

As mentioned, the film by *ErosErotica* demonstrating jelqing is not to be missed, and as said in the film, after the exercise the lad can reward himself with an orgasm, or save himself for his partner.

Stretching

Stretching is an alterative to jelqing but seems far less fun. The penis is wrapped in a towel, heated with hot water, and then pulled by the glans, *always* when soft. If hardness takes place, stop pulling, rewarm the penis until soft, and then go back to stretching.

Weights

Weights attached to the penis have been used since Greek times, and were used by Jews who clamped them on to what remained of their foreskins [*foreskins at that time were not totally cut off as today*]. The exposed glans was judged ugly by the Greeks, so in order for a Jew to participate in Greek exercises and in competitions his foreskin had to be restored.

One study suggests hanging 12 lbs from the penis for 15 minutes, repeated in 3 series. One can apparently do all-day hanging by attaching 1-2 lbs to a hanging device that is worn down the pant leg.

Hormones and Aphrodisiacs

These are the most sold hormones on the market, but the reader will have to investigate, on his own, whether they're of possible use to him, although studies repeatedly state that pills to nothing to increase the size of the phallus. This is how the companies that produce the hormones see themselves:

MaleExtra—enhances penis enlargement, promotes hardness, intensifies the orgasm and boosts the libido.

VigRx Plus—increases penis enlargement and harness, intensifies both stamina and orgasms.

Climinax—increases stamina and hardness.

The aim of the first great explorers was the find the Spice Islands, where magic pepper, ginger, saffron, cinnamon, cloves and nutmeg were found. Nutmeg was an aphrodisiac of choice, and found its way into medieval sex manuals as a way of boosting male libidos, but also a way to enlarge the phallus: ''A man who wants to make his member grand or fortify it for the coitus, must rub it before copulation with tepid water, until it gets red and extended by the blood flowing into it, in consequence of the heat; he must then anoint it with a mixture of honey and ginger, rubbing it in sedulously. Then let him join the woman; he will procure for her such pleasure that she objects to him getting off her again.'' A quote brought to us by Nigel Cliff.

Cock Rings

Cock rings are rubber donut-shaped devices that tightly encircle the penis at the base [or the penis and the balls]. They maintain an erection and give it a slight boost in size by cutting off the vein that carries blood out of the engorged dick, located on the upper surface of the penis, but does not influence the artery that brings blood in.

Piercing

''When Magellan exited the straits that now bare his name, he is said to have cried for joy. He was now in the Pacific, a stretch of water, in his mind, less in width than the Atlantic. He would discover that, in reality, it covered half the world, and he was already nearly out of food. Thanks to the Trade Winds, they made it to Guam three months later, although many men were dead from scurvy. They reached Cebu several months after that. Here Magellan became blood brothers with the Prince, both of whom mingled their blood in a bowl mixed with wine that they drank. Ravishing young girls were offered, virgins who had their vaginas enlarged from birth in order to accommodate men who inserted gold bolts through their penises, just under the glans. The tube of the bolts had a hole through which urine passed. The bolted penises were difficult to insert and they didn't allow rapid movements, meaning that intercourse lasted a very long time, even an entire day, and the men could pull out only when soft. The women claimed the bolts gave them ultimate pleasure.'' An extract from my book *Homosexual Warriors*.

The Prince Albert

The Prince Albert is a ring that extends from under the glans, through the urethra, and exits at the tip of the penis. Legend has it that Prince Albert used it to pull his penis upward, as Greek boys did in what was called infibulations [see the chapter on foreskins], in order for his dick to not be seen through his trousers [it was said to have been huge], a way of honoring his wife Victoria's modesty. [In the same way, when the South Kensington Museum received a full-sized copy of Michelangelo's *David* it had a special fig leaf of stone made, for use during visits of the queen.]

The piercing can be centered if the penis is circumcised; otherwise the piercing must be done off-center so that the foreskin can reposition itself [as I'm cut, I have no idea what this means]. The healing time can take from 4 weeks to 6 months [!]. Some users swear it enhances the sexual pleasure of both partners, others warn that in fellatio it can chip a tooth and provoke choking. They can be removed during sex.

Prince Albert piercing.

Hafada

The hafada is a piercing located anywhere on the skin of the scrotum.

Another example of male enhancement is brought to us by Nigel Cliff, one what intrigued the crew of Vasco da Gama's ships when they landed in India, the men instantly rock-hard at the view of Indian women. One noted a custom that allowed the women maximum coital felicity: ''Niccolò de' Conti had come across many shops run by women who sold strange objects, the size of a small nut and made of gold, silver, or brass, that tinkled like a bell. The men, he explained, before they take a wife, go to these women who cut the skin of the virile member in many places and put between the skin and the flesh as many as twelve of these bells, according to their pleasure. After the member is sewn up, it heals in a few days. This they do to satisfy the wantonness of the women: because of these swellings, or tumor, of the member, the women have great pleasure in coitus. The members of some men stretch way down between their legs so that when they walk they ring out and may be heard.''

THE ANATOMY OF THE BEAST

In a book on the phallus the beast has to be described, which I will do very briefly, based on the zones that offer the most pleasure.

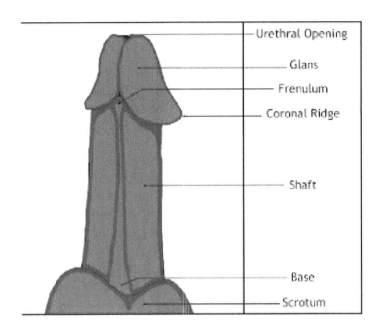

Urethral Opening

Glans

Frenulum

Coronal Ridge

Shaft

Base

Scrotum

The base of the penis shaft can be ringed with an elastic band which will allow the penis to fill with blood, but as the vein that carries the blood away from the shaft is located on the upper part of the shaft, it will be blocked. Blood will continue to enter but not to exit, which makes for a harder shaft, a slightly longer shaft, and a shaft that stays hard longer.

The head of the penis, or glans, is cut by a valley, the frenulum, a source of immense pleasure when stroked by fingers or tongue.

The length of a penis, flask, does not correspond to its length when hard, although a long flask penis is sought after when parading around the gym, and it does *suggest* triumphant length when hard. Apparently, the longest penis found by a doctor was 13.5 inches [34.3 cm], 6.26 inches around [15.9 cm].

Phalluses can be straight or curved, both erotically exciting in their own ways [offering a bit of diversity for Austrian women who have an average of 29 different males during their lifetimes].

A study of thousands of boys has shown that there is no difference in erect penis size from boys who are 17 compared to when they are 19, indicating that growth stops at age 17.

The purpose of the coronal ridge appears to be to encircle sperm deposited by a previous male and force it out of the vagina, the resulting vacant space filled with the new partner's semen. [I'm personally dubious, but there must be some biological reason for the phallus's arrowhead shape]. The deeper the thrust, the more ''foreign'' sperm will be removed.

FORESKINS

Porn star Al Parker had gone through the usual surgical disfigurement at birth, the loss of his foreskin, and throughout his life and films long, long minutes were dedicated to pulling, tonguing and manipulating the foreskin of the boys often chosen because they possessed one, his obsession with the loss of his natural right leading to its replacement, an operation wonderfully successful. In Greek times the exposed glans was considered so unaesthetic that a boy's foreskin was pulled forward and the tip tied shut. Some of the boys had the string from the foreskin attached to a string they wore around their waists, a method that stretched the penis upwards and fully exposed the balls. The string was called the *kynodesmē*, the leash for the dog. Circumcised Jews were not allowed to participate in Greek games, as said, because of the exposed glans. To overcome the ban the Jews attached weights to what remained of their foreskins, producing a new foreskin over time. Some resorted to surgery, but many died from the resulting infections.

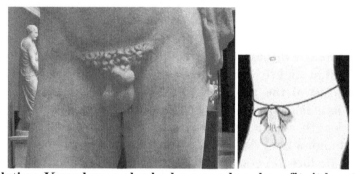

Infibulation. Kynodesme also had a secondary benefit: it lengthened the foreskins so that foreskins that didn't originally cover the entire glans, finally did.

The erotic view of boys and young men naked, aided by a climate that encouraged the dropping of clothing, made nude exercising and sports the enjoyable aspect of young men's daily activities, and older men came as spectators, talking affairs and politics while admiring pectorals and the curve of young buttocks. *Gymnos* from gymnasium means naked, and access to gymnasiums was forbidden to adults over 18, although Plato and Socrates had a dispensation, and for all of their talk of Platonic friendships, both used the renown of their schools to do far more than just talk.

Lads wore a chiton that fell to the thighs, shorter than today's kilts, and a slight lecherous breeze could do miracles in revealing a boy's hidden attributes. It was apparently not uncommon for a man to greet a youth by gently nudging his balls through the light tissue, and we have this from Aristophanes's *The Birds*: "You meet my son as he comes out of the gymnasium, all fresh from his bath, and you don't kiss him or feel his balls."

Parker changed the way men dressed, and during the '70s and '80s beards were often adopted, while mustaches became a must.

Little is known about his boyhood. His family was loving and he liked sports, baseball and swimming, and worked as a delivery boy. He discovered autoeroticism early but his favorite way of getting off was autofellation. By accident he came across an ad for Colt photos delivered through the mail, which he ordered. The sexual excitation when he saw the contents of the package made his sexual orientation crystal clear, if it hadn't been before then.

At age 17 his mother let him go to the Woodstock Festival in her Mustang convertible. The access to the concert was slow going because of the numerous cars and as he passed rivers and pools he was sexually stimulated by the sight of naked men and boys bathing to cool themselves off in the hot summer heat. At Woodstock the kids, on grass and other drugs, were having sex in the fields as if they were alone on the planet and Parker, who often retold the story to friends, had a perpetual erection, easily seen through his jeans, as by then his member was 9" long. Walking past a car he saw a guy stretched out inside with perfect six-pack abdominals, stone-hard pectorals, and totally nude. The guy kicked the door open and immediately went down on Parker when he sat beside him. It was Al's first uncut dick, the catalyst of his obsession. They both came, then and multiple times during the following days. Incredibly, when Al got home he found that his picture had been taken at Woodstock, and was on the Woodstock poster that later came out, making him an instant high-school celebrity. At any rate, one can hardly imagine a better entry into the gay world for a lad of 17 (4).

Al Parker had his foreskin restored, which can basically be done in several ways, surgery that transplants scrotal tissue to the penile shaft being one of them, and tugging that can stretch the foreskin back over the head of the penis. Tugging guarantees that there are nerve endings in the reconstructed foreskin, surgical intervention does not [details follow].

115 million Americans are said to be circumcised, 660 million worldwide, 83% of Americans were circumcised in the 1980s, 73% today, a practice so accepted that some doctors didn't even bother consulting a boy's parents; they just did it and put it somewhere in the bill. I personally saw my first uncut dick in the COPAR, a central gym attached to Parisian

universities. The massacre is declining, with the U.S. low of 30% on the West Coast [compared to 1.6% in Denmark].

Why circumcision became a national desecration is disputed: some researchers say it was thought to lessen masturbation, a typically American Puritan No-no. Some scientists claim that when the foreskin is not thoroughly cleaned it admits an odor that young boys find pleasurable and draws their attention to their penises, leading to masturbation. Others maintain that foreskins could cause cancer or minor infections if, again, the area was not sufficiently cleansed. Foreskins are thought by some doctors to favor herpes and other sexually transmitted diseases, and in 2014 the U.S. Center for Disease Control and Prevention *endorsed infant male circumcision*, something all medical institutions outside the United States categorically refute. [In Europe it has been admitted that circumcision could reduce urinary track infections by 1%, but this is countered by the number of hemorrhages, infections and even an occasional--if rare--death when a boy is circumcised.]

Legislation was passed in Germany, Finland, Denmark and Sweden declaring that circumcision, even religious--Jews and Muslims--is illegal because it violates a child's right to physical integrity and self-determination, a law disregarded by the above religions and not enforced by the countries. In Arab circumcision is called the ''purification'' and is not mentioned in the Koran, nor is it part of the five rules of Islam.

Some parents believe that boys with uncut dicks would be ridiculed in locker rooms, and so circumcision was a protection against harassment, while those who favor foreskins state that the only time a boy is harassed is when his dick is too small, this being pretty rare if one can judge from undercover videos taken in Marine locker rooms where *everyone* is small-- when flaccid, of course. [What takes place when the blood rushes there is, in many cases, utterly spectacular, and fascinating for women--and many men--to watch.]

The foreskin protects the head of the penis, and especially the sensitive frenulum, making sure that it remains sensitive, which is no longer the case when the foreskin is removed, meaning perhaps that a guy can have sex longer before cuming, but at what loss of pleasure, when one realizes that there are *20,000 nerves* destroyed when doctors remove the *15 square inches* for foreskin [in *adult* males]. Foreskins also hold in natural secretions which is great when jerking off, a natural source of lubrication, freeing the boy from alternatives like baby oil.

Foreskins make the penis look much longer, a huge advantage to locker-room athletes when all eyes are drawn to their members while they relate how well they screwed Suzy-Q the night before [''I made her cum three times,'' said one Marine filmed by a hidden camera]. All boys want to look their best when nude, and guys who have big dongs when hard, but look small when soft, gripe about still another of life's injustices.

Porn star Scott O'Hara (4) wrote this about foreskins: "My primary fetish: foreskin. I have one vivid memory of a foreskin from the my adolescent years--an older boys in the locker room whose penis was the most perfect torpedo I have ever seen, before or since. I only saw it once, but the memory is branded on my brain cells. The fact that he was one year older undoubtedly made it even more memorable. And yes, even at age fourteen, I knew without a moment's hesitation that I wanted to fall down and worship that hunk of meat [no, it wasn't huge--just very pretty]."

The mutilation of the human penis was practiced by the Egyptians in at least 4000 B.C., as witnessed by mummies dating from the period, and on the walls of tombs in Saqqara it is seen being performed on young boys, in paintings of exquisite beauty. Jewish Abraham circumcised himself at age 99, as well as the children he had before and afterwards, as his wife was only 90.

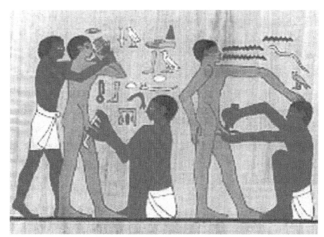

Egyptian circumcision originated with priests but was soon practiced on boys 13 and 14, and after the Vth Dynasty all the pharaohs were circumcised, state Bonnard and Schouman. Today circumcision is a clear violation of a boy's human rights, a disgusting mutilation ordered by ignorant parents and performed by doctors who want the additional fees.

The 20,000 nerves in the foreskin, enriched by a good supply of blood, add to sexual pleasure and the foreskin is a natural lubricator, adding also to sexual bliss, as well as protecting the glans from becoming dry and callused, thereby desensitizing it. One statistic has 73% of all American men circumcised [statistics very immensely], with San Francisco the heart of opposition to the disfigurement [although San Francisco was *for* circumcision during the gay plague because the foreskin was believed to facilitate the transfer of the disease].

FORESKIN RESTORATION

Jews were ''lightly'' circumcised, at times nearly only symbolically cut, which made the stretching of the existent foreskin infinitely easier and more rapid. Foreskins were of such esthetic beauty to the Greeks and Romans that they had laws against circumcision.

Today the battle wages between doctors who claim that foreskins are made of nerve-rich tissue and that circumcision is ''penile rape'', while others maintain that, in sensitivity, it makes no difference. As I've written, foreskins do cover 15 square inches, lots of which are made up of nerves. When erotically stimulated local nerves release nitric oxide to make the penile arteries open and allow blood to gush into the thousands of tiny sinusoid veins fanning out from the arteries, filling the foreskin and filling the phallus's central corpora cavernosa, the twin sponge-like chambers on either side of it. Meaning: no matter what doctors feel, it's obviously better to have the nerve ending in foreskins than it is to not have them.

The purpose of restoring one's foreskin is, first, aesthetics: the foreskin is a thing of immense beauty, and with its restoration a man's image of himself is vastly improved. He is whole again. Sexual stimulation is improved by a gain in sensitivity, and the new mobility, the gliding motion, is a boon to autoeroticism. Tugging methods can also lengthen the foreskins of those who have not been circumcised, for additional erotic effect. [There are a dozen tutorials on YouTube--in addition to the methods that follow-- that show step-by-step tugging techniques.]

Using only your hands, manually tug the skin under the corona up and over the glans--as far as possible, given the amount of foreskin you have left. In this way, over time, you will get enough skin in order to use a device you can wear under your clothes. Tension should be applied for 5 to 30 seconds at a time, then repeated.

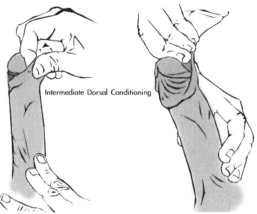

Intermediate Dorsal Conditioning

This method is followed by a second method in which an OK-grip if formed. It is pure jelqing:

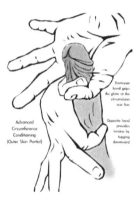

Dominant hand grips the glans at the circumcision scar line

Opposite hand provides tension by tugging downward

Advanced Circumference Conditioning (Outer Skin Partial)

The purpose is to induce mitosis [soon explained]. Once one has created some foreskin, one can pass to T-taping and/or a device, as explained elsewhere.

Some men manually tug 1 to 2 hours a day, every day. They tug for about 5 to 15 minutes during their shower. One can tug flaccid or erect, although it is easier to manually tug when erect.

Use as much tension as possible <u>without hurting yourself</u>. There must be no pain.

These two methods are followed by another, once you have some foreskin to grasp:

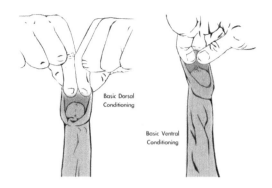

In this method you are focusing on the inner foreskin, tensioning those areas you wish to see grow, tugging the skin away from the glans.

This method is followed by a final method in which you have enough foreskin to grasp. You seize the end of the foreskin and pull it in the opposite direction to your other hand that has grasped the shaft in an OK-grip and is gently pulling to down towards the scrotum.

The above material was taken from RestoringForeskin.org.

Here we have additional drawings from another source, known simple as Doug's *Manual Methods of Foreskin Restoration*:

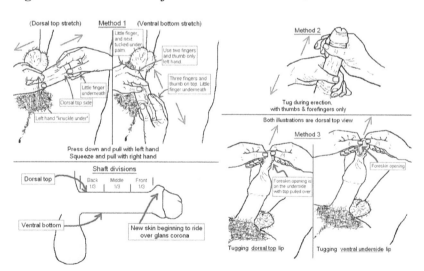

Surgery

One form of surgical restoration involves tissue from the scrotum. It is extremely expensive, $15,000 at the very least, and three operations are needed [if there are no complications, which there often are]. The shaft is denuded and inserted into scrotal tissue; 6 months later there is another surgery; six months later touch-up surgery; and even then only 60-70% of the operations are successful, although the esthetic results are rarely attained [there are apparently some men who claim to be satisfied].

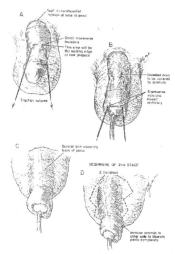

The purpose of this drawing is simple to give the reader an idea of what is to be avoided, as the outcome will be, in most cases, cosmetically unsatisfactory. If this weren't scary enough, scrotum hairs have to be eliminated, from the new foreskin, one by one. Most restoration groups advise against surgery, and are equally against surgery to lengthen and thicken the phallus.

Porn star Al Parker had his foreskin restored by Dr. Ira Sharlip. The operation consisted of making incisions around the penis to allow excess skin to be drawn forward. It was a huge success, the end product of which was an esthetic foreskin, as seen in Parker's highly erotic films. Parker, introduced as Drew Okun, his real name, went on t.v. to laud the surgery.

Tugging and mitosis

In tugging you are trying to induce mitosis in your remaining foreskin so it will grow more skin [in cell biology mitosis is a part of the cell cycle when replicated chromosomes are separated into two new nuclei. The cell membrane is divided into two new cells containing roughly equal shares of cellular components].

The Pondus Judaeus

The Pondus Judaeus was a bronze sheath used to expand the foreskin when the foreskin had not been fully excised. [No detailed description or illustration exist.] It was to avoid this type of restoration that the Jews resorted to complete circumcision and not token circumcision, which had been the case.

T-Tape [tape only] and Tape with weights

Hospital-type tape pulls the skin forward:

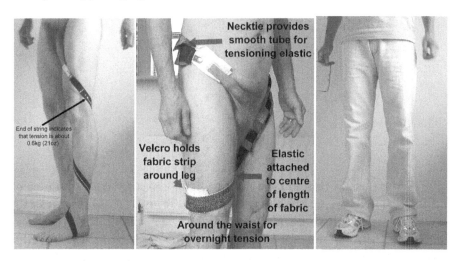

The tape can also be attached to weights and can be worn for **24 hours.** If the user feels any pain he must stop, as this should not, in any way, hurt.

DTR [duel tension restoration]

A device, like a cone or plastic shell, is placed over the glans. The skin is pulled onto the device. Tape is applied to keep the skin in place. The device is then pulled by using a rubber band or a weight. *But it's entirely dicey if you haven't much foreskin left to work with.*

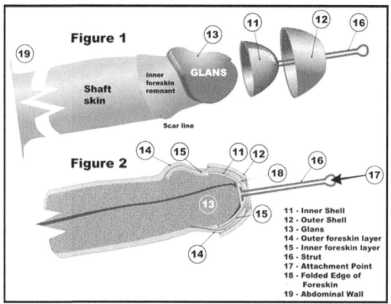

Figure 1

Figure 2

11 - Inner Shell
12 - Outer Shell
13 - Glans
14 - Outer foreskin layer
15 - Inner foreskin layer
16 - Strut
17 - Attachment Point
18 - Folded Edge of
     Foreskin
19 - Abdominal Wall

Picture and following how-to from *Wikipedia*.

The device without tape:
A device, such as a cone, bell or shell, is placed over the glans
Skin is pulled onto the device
The skin is covered with a flexible gripping cap
Tension is applied by pulling the device.

The device with tape:
A device, such as a cone, bell or shell, is placed over the glans
Skin is pulled onto the device
Tape is applied to keep the skin in place
The device is then pulled using a rubber band or has a weight to apply tension.

The reader may want to consult Tug Ahoy for other methods, and Net sites devoted to other DTR devices, as well as TLG Tugger and TLC-X, the purpose of this chapter being simply to put the victim of foreskin profanation on the right track to foreskin restoration.

Sculptor Michael Dulin has spent a part of his life fighting against what he calls the atrocity of circumcision. As a victim himself, he had his restored. Married, he was in the hospital visiting his wife and their first child when he met a man who had just videotaped his boy's circumcision and was ''bragging about how the kid screamed and blood spurted everywhere.''

Dulin's foreskin restoration took four years, but, he says, was only a facsimile of a foreskin, one that could never replace the 60,000 nerve endings [his number] cut along with the 15 square inches of lost skin.

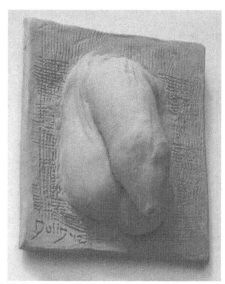

Michael Dulin's terracotta foreskin.

The procedure may take several years, depending on the amount of skin available to expand. It also depends on the man's commitment, the techniques used, and the body's degree of plasticity [its capacity to be altered]. In some cities there are support groups, a great way of making new friends. The chief support group is NORM, the National Organization of Restoring Men. [A story circulated that the founder of NORM, Wayne Griffiths, wore ball bearings attached to his foreskin by tape, one of which became detached and fell to the floor during a meeting. At the time his foreskin was said to have surpassed is glans by ¾ of an inch, and was responsible for a huge gain in sensitivity and sexual enjoyment.]

Once the foreskin has been restored through some form of tugging, a slight surgical intervention can reduce the size of the opening, so that the finished reconstruction produces a nearly normal-appearing prepuce [otherwise the foreskin will slide away from the glans, which is not the effect desired. That said, nothing stops a guy from continuing until he has a very long foreskin, which will then stay in place over the glans].

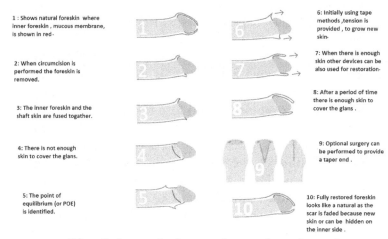

1 : Shows natural foreskin where inner foreskin , mucous membrane, is shown in red .

2: When circumcision is performed the foreskin is removed.

3: The inner foreskin and the shaft skin are fused togather.

4: There is not enough skin to cover the glans.

5: The point of equilibrium (or POE) is identified.

6: Initially using tape methods ,tension is provided , to grow new skin.

7: When there is enough skin other devices can be also used for restoration.

8: After a period of time there is enough skin to cover the glans .

9: Optional surgery can be performed to provide a taper end .

10: Fully restored foreskin looks like a natural as the scar is faded because new skin or can be hidden on the inner side .

The slight surgical operation spoken about above.

Foreskin/prepuce reconstruction/restoration will never replace the lost foreskin, which contained nerve endings, muscles and blood vessels, all of which hugely added to one's sexual sensations, although these functions can be recuperated *to some degree.* Restoration can *enhance* the sexual experience, and restore a man's feeling of wholeness. The benefactor is no longer totally mutilated.

Restoring the foreskin and lengthening the phallus has produced a whole new industry, and at this very moment tens of thousands of men may be using devises for said reconstruction.

KING TESTOSTERONE

Testosterone is basically produced in the testicles and has two effects, one called anabolic and includes muscle and bone mass and strength. The second is androgenic and changes a boy's appearance into that of a man: a deeper voice; penis and testicle size; body hair--pubic, facial and underarm. It stimulates the libido. It's what makes us horny, what gives us an erection and the body muscle to put it to use. It is the god virility.

The brain is responsible for the orgasm, but testosterone develops everything a man wants to visually see: a phallus pointed straight up from a full bush of pubic hair, biceps and pectorals, body odor and the oily shine to the skin.

Foreplay and porn movies greatly increase testosterone levels, levels that fall significantly after two to three years of marriage, but not in boys who continue to play the field. In that it's the fountain of youth, one that extends far longer in men who remain single. Testosterone levels can be augmented by a decrease in weight, because fat cells synthesize an enzyme that converts testosterone into a female hormone. Licorice apparently increases testosterone levels, along with tuna, grapes, pomegranate, venison, garlic, honey, milk, eggs and cabbage.

A motor needs to be turned every day. If not, it will eventually fail. With age and the lessening of testosterone a lad's lust diminishes. If one doesn't insist on turning the motor, he will lose his will to do so, and with it a huge part of himself will die forever. Go to the Net and the porn channel you prefer. The heat will build, the lust and desire for the orgasm will soon have you panting, and although the orgasm will lack a bit in intensity, and you may not be able to perform six times a day as when you were an adolescent, nor cum in a minute and be ready to cum again in half-an-hour, your virility will nonetheless still be intact, and will gratefully award you with a moment of pleasure, a moment that is perhaps the very first real comfort, the very first real happiness, in an adolescent boy's life.

[Although in Paris in 1753 one boy was recorded to have killed himself when he had intercourse 18 times in 10 hours.]

PRE-CUM

Pre-cum is emitted by the penis head when sexually aroused. It is an acid-neutralizer and lubricant, and as such far more enjoyable to men who are not circumcised, especially with foreplay activities with a partner(s) and for autoeroticism. It is produced by the Cowper's glands [bulbourethral glands] and the glands of Littre, and contains some spermatozoa, which makes *coitus interruptus* dicey as a replacement for condoms in preventing pregnancies. The amount issued varies hugely, and its sight is erotic because it means that the partner is playing his/her role in arousal.

SEMEN

The testicles produce testosterone. Hugely increased during puberty, it deepens the voice, creates body hair and makes desire overwhelming, to the point that a boy will bed anything, and then kick himself in the butt for doing so, once he's had release and he sees with what he's just made love [in *The Last Picture Show* (the book) boys did it with calves]. The urge with James Boswell was so strong he contracted the clap 17 times in 9 years [gonorrhea], and Walter of *My Secret Life* had the clap again and again, despite being laid up for weeks each time, the price of his need for sex. Luckily today's boys have functioning rubbers for protection. During Victorian times boys plunged into the Thames in winter as a method of lessoning desire, the same desire that will propel men to cheat on the wives they adore. Herodotus tells us that when women died in Egypt their husbands would not deliver the bodies to be mummified until several days later, to avoid their being violated by embalmers. Byron had what he called full intercourse with 200 lads in Athens, and only then declared himself f*cked-out in a letter to a friend. Hickman relates that boys are regularly taken to hospital emergencies when having unsuccessfully copulated with vacuum cleaners. Portnoy f*cked the family dinner liver and then ate it along with the others, and de Sade and the star of *American Pie* had limitless imaginations.

Semen can spurt from a distance of an inch or two to eight feet, the ejaculate usually less than a spoonful. It is produced in the scrotal sac which is made of the thinnest tissue on the body. 70 million spermatozoa are turned out daily and make up around 2.5% of the ejaculate, the remaining fluids from the prostate and seminal glands. A finished spermatozoa takes from 2 to 3 months to produce [!]. Hickman tells us that sperm lasts ''a month in the staging area, two days inside a woman's body, perhaps two minutes on the sheets,'' and 300,000,000 sperm, united, would make one grain of sand. The head of the spermatozoa has the DNA, and is capped by enzymes that allow it to pierce the ovum. One ejaculate could fertilize every woman on the planet [or so it's consistently said].

Some men, Howard Hughes among them (4), believe that ingesting semen is the secret elixir to eternal youth and boundless energy. It isn't, but still incomplete scientific research indicates that it has tremendous health value, and lapping it up from a boy's solid abs is, in addition, highly erotic.

As we've seen, semen can be in such abundance as to fill rivers, the Tigris and Euphrates, the Nile and Ganges. An ejaculation can fly well over a boy's head, or end up in rivers and lakes over abs and chest, as well as just coat the upper fingers of the o.k.-grip that brought him up and over.

Hormones released during intercourse lower blood pressure, decrease bad cholesterol, greatly lessen stress, can diminish the risk of heart attacks and, according to Hickman, an orgasm can be ''as much as ten times more effective than Valium.'' It is also the best way to send a guy into the arms of welcoming Morpheus.

Research indicates that a male shown a picture of a naked female and two naked males will produced more vigorous and more abundant spermatozoa than if he is shown a picture of three naked females, because he would find himself in completion with the males to fertilize the female [and the possibility that he may be partially gay...?].

The longer the penis the closer to the ovum, which would seem to enhance fertilization, but researchers insist on sperm quality and vigor as the prime factors, not penile length.

A boy at times suffers through the negligence and even, perhaps, the brutality of his father, and no matter how intelligent the boy is, and despite the education he receives, nothing will ever erase the emptiness and hurt he'll carrying in his heart and in the pit of his stomach throughout the rest of his life. Yet had his father not deposited his semen--because that was what everyone else was doing--and have a son--because it was the expected ritual of manhood--in a word, had he abstained, then I wouldn't be here to write these words. That is the dichotomy of to be or not to be.

FOREPLAY

It's true that men favor quick and erotic ejaculations, greatly inspired by natural settings, forests, lakes and beaches, or humping along some dark alley, especially at night, when all cats are indeed grey. A pull at two short ribbons freed Renaissance boys for action, and later codpieces were said to not have been attached at the top in order to allow rapid access when urinating and wenching.

Yet unhurried sex, called foreplay, exists too, and in this homosexuals are world-class champions, as they intimately know what turns the other on, which is what turns them on, and the more they apply themselves, the more they'll be ''applied'' in return. In my book *Hustlers* I mention the case of Alex Garrett and the first time he was reamed, the surprise in his eyes captured on film, a lad who claimed to have been heterosexual and unaware of even the existence of a tongue in such a place.

Guys today automatically expect chicks to go down on them, and more and more boys return the favor by going down on girls, some guys seemingly loving to do so, while others prefer minimal service with fingers substituting for tongues. Historically cunnilingus has had a bad press, in part because it wasn't a virile exercise, in part because it was deemed unclean, especially in ages of little bathing. But *all* homosexuals want to take out the as-yet unseen object of curiosity, the phallus, straining against the fabric of jeans and briefs, and mouth it.

Nipples become erect like the phallus and as such are eminently erotic, as are underarms begging to be nuzzled with the tongue. Errol Flynn (3) invited boys on his boat *Sirocco*, and those he wanted back were given roles in his films. One lad was to play a captive with his wrists tied high above his head, his armpits in full view. Judged too hairy by the director, he ordered them trimmed. Flynn stepped in, proclaiming that there was nothing sexier than the lad's two pussies.

Pussies, underarms may not be; sexy they are.

If a gay can get a straight to submit to a massage, he's won the day. Otherwise gay sex does not involve Tantric preparation, but is more direct

[Tantric sexual exercises often forgo orgasm entirely, in favor of self control, where, for most men, the aim of the game *is* the orgasm]. In Greece a boy expected a man to walk up and gentle caress his balls through the tissue of his chiton, and as stated earlier, Aristophanes has a man in one of his plays complain to another that he neglected his son in not kneading his attributes when they'd met on the street. Today such directness could only take place in saunas and gay discos, but it shows that we've invented nothing, sexually, and that our ancient forefathers may have had it far better.

A study of 2,300 women in Prague concluded that what interested them was the duration of intercourse, not foreplay. Whereas for homosexual men foreplay is intercourse in another form, and an orgasm, while standing, kissing and mutually manipulating each other's sword, can be every bit as powerful as ejaculating through intercourse.

Nipples are of huge erotic importance, as said, and some men, like Tyron Power, could have an orgasm simply by having their nipples caressed with fingers or tongue [although he craved anal sex, and he would continually spur the top on by telling him how great he was, and how much pleasure he was giving].

Boys without pubic hair are not sexually exciting, as far as I'm concerned, but shaved balls allow a clearer, more erotic view during foreplay and makes licking and sucking them far easier. The slit at the head of the phallus, as well as the frenulum, are of great sensitivity, and a little additional foreplay with the tongue will prove to your partner that you know what you're doing, and may encourage him to return the favor.

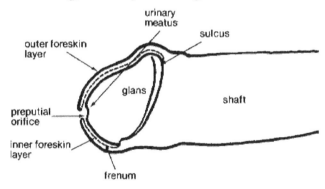

[The sulcus is simply the groove between glans and shaft. The frenulum (or frenum) is the extremely sensitive skin on the underside of the shaft, attaching the glans to the shaft.]

You can read articles in the hundreds of magazine that advise women on exactly how to please hubby and/or boyfriend, you can search through them until the cows come home, and you will find nothing on reaming. A pleasure at least equal to nipple and dick sucking, reaming is mostly unknown among heterosexuals. A few magazines will touch on the male G-spot, the prostrate, and in skirted terms tell girls the ins-and-outs of how to put pressure on the perineum [located between the anus and balls, pressure there can retard orgasm, giving gals longer time in the saddle]. As mentioned elsewhere, straight gay-for-pay porn star Alex Garrett was filmed showing shock during his first reaming, shock that soon changed into Nirvana-level bliss. Straight boys don't expect to get reamed, gay boys dream of it, part-and-parcel of the mounting orgasm.

AUTOEROTICISM

The most common masturbation technique, *Wikipedia* informs us, ''is by gripping and sliding the foreskin back and forth [a reason the foreskin must not be circumcised] and by moving the hand up and down the shaft. This type of stimulation is typically all that is required to achieve orgasm and ejaculation. The speed of the hand motion will vary, although it is common for the speed to increase as ejaculation nears and for it to decrease during the ejaculation itself.'' Perfect. Circumcised males need a lubricant such as spit, which is tragically incomplete compared to Nature's original gift.

The word itself may come from *manus* [hand] + *stupare* [to defile] or *mas* [penis] + *turbatio* [to excite]. [Onanism must not be confused with masturbation, as it is *coïtus interruptus*, ejaculation outside the vagina to avoid pregnancies.]

''Lying face down on a comfortable surface such as a mattress or pillow, the penis can be rubbed against it. This technique may include the use of a simulacrum, or artificial vagina,'' continues *Wikipedia*.

''There are many other variations on male masturbation techniques. Men may also rub or massage the glans, the rim of the glans. Some men place both hands directly on their penis during masturbation, while others may use their free hand to fondle their testicles, nipples, or other parts of their body. The nipples are erogenous zones, and vigorous stimulation of them during masturbation usually causes the penis to become erect more quickly than it would otherwise. Some may keep their hand stationary while pumping into it with pelvic thrusts in order to simulate the motions of sexual intercourse. A few extremely flexible males can reach and stimulate their penis with their tongue or lips, and so perform autofellatio.''

Wikipedia, no prude, goes on:

''The prostate gland is one of the organs that contributes fluid to semen. As the prostate is touch-sensitive, some directly stimulate it using a well-lubricated finger or dildo inserted through the anus into the rectum.

''Mutual masturbation is a sexual act where two *or more people* stimulate themselves or one another sexually, usually with the hands. It is practiced by people of all sexual orientations, and can be part of a full repertoire of sexual activity. It may be used as foreplay, or as an alternative to sexual penetration" [my emphasis].

"Frequency of masturbation is determined by many factors, e.g., one's resistance to sexual tension, hormone levels influencing sexual arousal, sexual habits, peer influences, health and one's attitude to masturbation formed by culture." End of article.

Incredibly, the only statistics concerning masturbation date from Kinsey, 60 years ago, meaning they are meaningless to our Internet generation. Today boys openly masturbate seated before their computers, careless of the presence of other males, an intimacy unheard of in past generations.

In 2009 the UK joined the Netherlands in encouraging daily masturbation as healthful, mindboggling when one considers the heinous reputation of "self-abuse" a few years back, one that continues in most other countries in the world, many of which continue to imprison homosexuals. In a Health Service leaflet in Sheffield entitled *Pleasure* one finds the slogan: *An orgasm a day keeps the doctors away.* It encourages the young to delay losing their virginity, a way of preventing unwanted pregnancies and diseases.

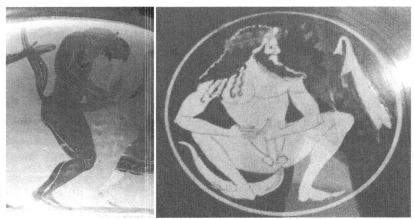

Satyrs – Greek krater – 550 B.C.

Autoeroticism is practiced by married men who generally have to conceal the fact, and by gays too in a relationship. It is a pleasant alternative, and as a man never leaves the house without his equipment, it can be performed absolutely anywhere when one feels the urge. In high school and at the university, especially in the library, when aroused, I needed only to move the eraser of my pencil over my buttoned levis fly, hidden by the table, to produce nearly instant ecstasy, *and* release from stress, *and* a welcomed time-out.

Autoeroticism is known to relieve depression and is said to increase one's self esteem, a far cry from my youth, as I write in my autobiography: ''The solution--oh so simple--consisted of keeping my hands out of the vicinity of the troubling area. Three nights after promising Mother and God I would never do it again, I had only to rub--of so minutely, *à peine*, just the tiniest little bit--the extended pouch of his jockeys five harmless times against the bed sheets to bring on a heavenly bliss with full angelic and choral accompaniment. The resulting mess would not have pleased my mother who found me the cleanest of lads, but if this was madness, I was ready for the asylum. The discovery of this innocent stroking of cotton against cotton as-if-so-help-me-God-I-didn't-know-what-was-going-on was, as the French say, *le pied*, their expression for ecstasy.'' (1)

A 1997 study reveals that frequent autoeroticism decreases the risk of heart attacks and it seems to lower blood pressure. That said, ''real sex'' is a better cardio-vascular workout, still another study affirms. A 2008 study at Tabriz Medical University states that frequent autoeroticism reduced swollen nasal blood vessels, rendering breathing easier.

The Greeks had no sexual hang ups and the birth of Aphrodite was due to Eros playing with himself, as in this extract from by book *TROY*:

"How were you born, marvelous Eros?" inquired Eos. "It's been so long since I left school that I've totally forgotten the History of the Beginning of Time."

"My parents," began Eros, eager to take the stage, "were Mother Desire and Father Deviation, two old gods dethroned by the new ones. All I remember is awaking in the middle of a pile of egg shells where the ocean laps against the shore." In his mind's eye he saw the long crescent beach with its tepid sands and lucent waters. His birth had been a moment of such divine ecstasy that he carried its sweet imprint throughout the whole of his eventful, carefree life.

"And at birth you found yourself completely on your own?" asked Helios.

"Yes, and as a god I was full-grown when only nine days old. I was very curious and since I was alone, I had only myself to play with. One day, therefore, as I was taking in the warmth of a brilliant afternoon and pursuing solitary amusement in the hollow of some rocks a few feet above the sea, I gave myself up to the most voluptuous of feelings, and low and behold from the place where my seed splattered upon the crystal waters rose up the most beautiful of women, naked and enthroned in a scallop shell. She rode on the foam of little wavelets that placed her ever so gently upon the sand. We immediately became great friends and discovered that we had a good deal in common: I, Eros, god of Passion and she, Aphrodite-- for such was her name--the goddess of Love. And as you know, we were made it hit-it-off and hit-it-off we did and always have."

Brought up by religious Tartuffes in Salt Lake City, I'll never forget my introduction to self-abuse: "On the Sunday in question a visiting bishop came into our all-male quorum to give us a little talk on sex, an unnerving proposition because the boys could not see what good a bishop could possible have to say on the subject. The bishop, in his early twenties, was stooped and sparrow chested, bad form for a people whose creed was the Body is the Temple of the Spirit. If that was his temple, a gnat resided within. His face was chinless and sunfish narrow, and in his eyes burned the fire of martyrs. The way to damnation, he told us right off, passed through wicked hands. At the university, he went on, he had had a roommate who openly aroused himself on the adjoining bed. But the bishop had been there with a handy yardstick to whack the boy when the Devil got into those pouncing fingers. Bending over us like a bloodless Ichabod Crane, he spewed visions of bodies rotting in hell and brains open cesspools to death maggots. The boys shrank back as much from the ejected spit and clots of foam at the corners of his razor-thin liver-colored lips as from fear of the contagion of his own personal madness. Those boys, so bright and beautiful, wormed their backs into the plywood seats, a scorching heat burning into necks and ears, their throats so dry they had to cough to swallow. We who survived thanks to that sin, we who could stay the strain of continence because of it, who could overcome the pressures of exams, of growing up, of *being* thanks to it, we who would one day have families of our own, build our country, *die* for it, we were being warped by this shell of a human being whose inanities we swallowed. Terror was indeed catching, and we fell victim to it" (1). This will give today's generation an idea of what boys then went through.

A boy openly masturbating on a beach in Sweden in 1213 was found innocent of all charges of indecency [the world will never catch up with Sweden on sexual freedoms].

In 2009 the Spanish region of Extremadura circulated a leaflet in a whopping €14,000 campaign that encouraged "sexual self-exploration and self-pleasure" from age 14 to 17!

Masturbation marathons have gone global, and May has been consecrated as Masturbation Month. British Channel 4 sponsored Wank Week.

In David Bret's *Errol Flynn* we learn that Flynn had a jack-off room in his home that gave onto a bedroom on the ground floor through a one-way mirror in the flooring. He chose the best-looking boys and girls and gave them the use of the bedroom while he and his pals, among them David Niven, bunched around, jerking off while the couples screwed below. Both Niven and Flynn had lives of incredible interest before they'd become stars.

Luckily Niven left us two books he wrote, *The Moon's a Balloon* and *Bring on the Empty Horses* that are simply wonderful (3).

Diogenes recommended autoeroticism because it was easily available and inexpensive, "If only one could satisfy one's hunger by rubbing one's stomach!"

For the Hebrews, who needed a big population, autoeroticism was a crime, and for Christianity a graver mortal sin than adultery. Even during the Enlightenment a man's semen was deemed finite, and so autoeroticism was a wasteful loss.

Once masturbation was found scientifically responsible for every physical ill known to man [due to a quack doctor, Samuel-Auguste Tissot, who condemned it in 1758], the resultant panic was the catalyst for a huge increase in circumcision, thought to deaden the head of the penis through its constant exposure, thusly lessoning one's urge to fondle it.

Incredibly, Freud maintained that only men, not women, practiced autoerotism, and that the whole thing was "infantile".

As homosexuals are obsessed by the genitals, they have made the circle jerk an erotic form of art, the pleasant memory of which is part of nearly every heterosexual's boyhood as well.

Whereas Jean-Jacque Rousseau found autoerotism "a dangerous supplement," the philosopher Denis Diderot wrote, in 1782, "It is a need and a sweet thing. It is a call from Nature to help it, and although we will not provoke it, let us lend it a helping hand, occasionally. I see only foolish, wasted pleasure in denying it." Diderot went on to confess: "My father's page boys taught me through kindness." For the Marquis de Sade, imprisoned for 30 years, autoerotism was the supreme pleasure: "He was jerking off. I watched the voluptuous sensation carrying him entirely out of himself, his moans, his groans, his strokes as he reached the very last stages of pleasure, and I saw his tool spill sperm in the same vase I'd just filled."

Psychiatrist and sexologist Philippe Brenot, author of *In Praise of Masturbation*, brings us this quote from Apollinaire, *The Debauched Hospodar*, 1907, "He started to masturbate them [2 girls], each with one hand, while they were exciting his cock." And on the Orient Express Apollinaire was relieved by his manservant: "Cornaboeux's fingers delicately unbuttoned the prince's trousers. They took hold of the delirious penis which on all accounts justified the famous couplet by Alphonse Allais: 'The exciting vibration of trains/Slides desire into the marrow of our loins.'"

Writer Michel Tournier wrote *The Meteors*: "The brain provides the sexual organ with an imaginary object. This object rests with the hand to embody it. The hand is the ideal partner. Like an actor the hand plays the role it is given, but its masterpiece is masturbation. There it becomes at will either a penis or a vagina.'' Guillaume Fabert wrote in *Self-portrait of an Erection*, masturbation ''is to sex what aspirin is to medicine: *panacea*.''

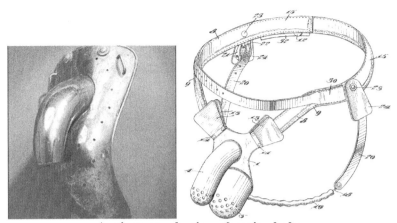

Anti-masturbation chastity belts.

The puritan John Kellogg was in charge of a mental asylum where masturbation among the inmates gave him the idea of inventing a food that would lessen sexual desire. He and his brother therefore invented Kellogg Cornflakes.

CONDOMS

As a sign of the times, the Swiss produce a condom for boys 12 to 14 called HOTSHOT [super name!], which has a diameter of 1.7 inches compared to normal-sized condoms of 2 inches. The Germans produce YOUNG LOVE with a diameter of 1.9 inches for the same age group. Both are as long as normal condoms, 7.4 inches.

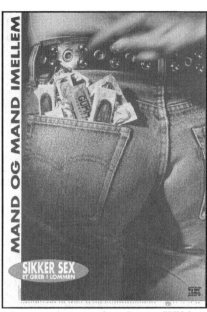

Condoms, picture thanks to *Wikipedia*.

Due to the usual religious nonsense and the feeling that one should be punished for lubricious activities, America was the only country that didn't provide condoms for its troops in W.W. I, and even Freud was against them because they reduced sexual pleasure. Casanova, on the other hand, was a user during the late 1700s, employing condoms from animal intestines that covered the glans and were called caps. Their immorality, expense and the ignorance of the lower classes made their use rare, but the upper classes could find them in the 1800s in pubs, barbershops and *theaters*. Some hospitals during the American Civil War refused to treat syphilis sufferers because they got what they deserved for their lack of morality.

Lambskin condoms prevented pregnancies but the pores were too large to stop sexually transmitted diseases. Today lambskin condoms-- thought to be "close to the real thing"--are still produced but are much more expensive.

Germany was the first country to provide condoms for its troops in W.W. I but banned them in W.W. II as boys were needed for future cannon fodder. America finally caught up in W.W. II with films showing soldiers the ravages of sexually transmitted diseases, although the accepted method of control was keeping the offender "in your pants".

Thanks to the invention of vulcanization by Goodyear in 1844, condoms, as thick as bicycle inner tubes, were produced in 1855. Hand dipped over penis-shaped molds, they were replaced by latex in the 1920s and by automation in the 1930s. Latex condoms mustn't be used with butter, margarine, baby oil, cooking oil, skin and suntan lotions. Sizes go from "snug" to "magnum". Particularly cautious wearers "double bag", two condoms at once, with perhaps less feeling, but otherwise Why not?

Los Angeles County forbade pornographic films that didn't use condoms, the result being the expatriation of production outside the county limits. Personally I hate to see guys condomless before action and then miraculously wearing condoms during intercourse. On the other hand, watching someone putting on a condom is, for me, the height of eroticism.

While 89% of Americans believe in God, only 9% say He plays a role in their daily lives. Likewise, although many religions are against the use of condoms, 80% of American parents want their children educated in their use during sex-ed classes.

Other benefits of condoms come through their use in protecting the muzzles of guns from the elements, and their value in delaying the ejaculation of rapid shooters, due to their [very slightly] dulling of sensation.

On French t.v. a boy [beautiful!] was interviewed about whether he used condoms. He said, seriously, that he observed a girl a certain time before arriving at the conclusion as to use a condom or not. I'm certain that such an attitude is widely shared, meaning that diseases--among the most horrifying--still have a bright future.

Durex does the research, Trojan condoms rake in the dough [which means that few out there know that the Trojans had been massacred at Troy (12)]. The name is genial anyway, as are the names of Trojan rubbers, Ultra Ribbed, Magnum XL, Warm Sensation, accounting for 70% of the market, 4 times runner-up Durex. Like the Marlboro Man, name is everything, and what guy isn't dying to try on an Ultra Ribbed, even if it's only to try it out with his hand?

W.W. I saw an explosion in the sale of condoms, to European armies, as the United States forces refused to supply them to their soldiers, as said, to hell with the epidemic of venereal diseases that broke out, and in the States themselves even pharmacies refused to stock them, back then, and bars made a killing out of backroom sales.

Minos, king of Crete, ejaculated sperm rich in scorpions and serpents, and was thusly forced to wear a condom made from a goat bladder in order to have intercourse. Romans had condoms made from goat bladders and pig guts, while during the Middle Ages condoms from animal bladders were considered implements of the Devil, and the user was burned at the stake. Under Henri III his mother Catherine de' Medici allowed condoms as a method for fighting syphilis, condoms already in use in Italy for the same reason. Condoms were attributed to the English who claimed that a knight, Sir Condom, Charles II's doctor, invented them, at the time called "gallant sacs", although the word may have, in reality, come from the Italian *condere*, to hide/protect.

ANAL SEX

One of the surprises I've had in watching porno on the Net is the incredible intensity of an orgasm through anal sex, showing men who beg for penetration, and are clearly more excited and vociferous during this form of lovemaking than the boy who is doing the drilling, the top. Although the prostate is a vital center in male orgasms when only the phallus is stimulated, penetration and direct stimulation of the prostate itself by the inserted phallus [or fingers or sex toy] is said to provoke a deeper orgasm, more widespread and intense, longer-lasting, far more ecstatic than when the phallus alone is stimulated. Some researchers believe the prostate is similar to the gland connected to the female G-spot.

Thanks to the Net one clearly follows the preparations that make a lad want penetration, and as some boys prefer the role of top, it is a win-win situation. Otherwise, the answer is to flip-flop, each male taking his turn.

Men can achieve orgasm exclusively through anal sex, with no stimulation whatsoever applied to the phallus of the bottom.

ORGASM

From the Greek ὀργασμός, meaning excitement + swelling + climax, it is euphoric pleasure caused by the stimulation of the phallus, autoerotically or with a partner(s). An orgasm increases in speed and intensity, beginning at the anal sphincter and traveling to the top of the phallus, a neuromuscular bliss that is unstoppable once begun. It lasts an average 10-15 seconds and occasionally can go on and on, up to 30 seconds.

Sperm is transmitted from the testicles into the prostate and seminal vesicles, then ejected as semen. With age the length of the orgasm is lessened, as is the amount of semen, but the intensity of the pleasure continues on.

A 1997 study in the *British Medical Journal* followed 918 men, aged 45-59, for 10 years. There was a reduction in heart attacks/stroke for those who had orgasms three or more times a week.

Boys can have six orgasms daily, and there's no reason why they shouldn't [although it's surprising, in interviews, to hear boys say that they often go weeks without]. There are two examples of men who believed that the loss of semen weakened them, to the point that Prince Aly Khan, who had made love to thousands of women, allowed himself two orgasms a week, and King Ibn-Saud of Saudi Arabia had had sex with women from age 11, sleeping with three different women every night, but limited himself to a single orgasm.

On the other hand, Indian Maharajas believed that sperm became rancid like milk and butter if left to accumulate. They had a woman hired to evacuate the semen within a maximum time of half-an-hour, either by offering herself or by masturbating him. The woman was otherwise obliged to remain chaste all her life. This took place when it was judged that the Maharaja was not coupling often enough with his wives.

Jewels, especially diamonds and emeralds, were thought to have aphrodisiac powers and Maharajas wore them during their crowning in order to keep his phallus erect. The obligation of maintaining an erection was later replaced by a symbolic belt of precious stones.

The countries apparently most satisfied with their sex lives are, in order, Switzerland, Spain, Italy, Brazil, Greece and Holland [ratings vary from one study to another]. A Durex study shows that the Greeks have sex the most often, 164 times a year, followed by Brazil, Poland and Russia. Greek men have 10 different sex partners throughout their lifetimes, while Greek women have 28! Austrian men come in first with 17 sex partners, while Austrian women have 29 different men.

TWO KEY HORMONES: DOPAMINE AND PROLACTIN

Dopamine drives us to have sex, as well as pushing us to do other activities which in turn trigger increases in dopamine, such as gambling and overeating [because high-fat and sugary foods, like ice cream, produce surges of dopamine]--*and* pornography.

After orgasms an ''off'' switch kicks in, putting on the brakes, caused by the hormone prolactin.

Dopamine pushes a guy to cum at all costs, prolactin makes him roll over and go to sleep, giving the next guy in line his chance. The woman is still ready for more, an assurance that she'll end up being fertilized by the most valiant and hardy of the semen she receives, as it's believed that only the strongest of men's sperm will be first to hit the target.

Gorgeous Douglas Fairbanks Jr. stated that during the sex act Laurence Olivier was as hot as a potato, but an iceberg immediately afterwards, refusing even a parting kiss--a man obviously hypersensitive to dopamine rushes, followed by excessive levels of prolactin.

HISTORY'S PHALLUS SUPER STUDS

History is full of men rumored to have been huge and to have enjoyed countless women, Warren Beatty who may have had 12,000, Porfirio

Rubirosa was said to have had 11'' that he shared with Marilyn Monroe, Jayne Mansfield, Zsa Zsa Gabor, *et al.*; Toulouse-Lautrec and Milton Berle. I would like to bring several men to the reader's attention, Giulio Romano, François I, Casanova, Byron, Valentino and Rubirosa, ending with a man who had had them all, Howard Hughes.

Giulio Romano
1499 – 1546

Raphael opened his own workshop with, says Vasari, fifty apprentices and assistants, one of whom was Caravaggio, among whom were his lovers, Giulio Romano and Gianfrancesco Penni. Thanks to these men Raphael was able to produce an amazing number of paintings. They all looked as though they had come from the hand of the master, but in reality many cooks had been involved. Raphael was especially noted as someone who would take over the techniques of others, incorporating any and all external influences. He was also a perfect collaborator, establishing peaceful relations between men of extremely varied characters. After Raphael's death Giulio Romano and Gianfrancesco Penni continued his workshop, their inheritance from Raphael.

Romano was Raphael's star student, whom he taught with ''tender loving care'' Vasari inform us. He soon mastered Raphael's techniques, from the mixing of colors to the secrets of perspective. Romano was not only intelligent and a quick study, he was ''inventive, affable, gracious and had the very finest manners,'' continues Vasari. Raphael would prepare paintings, drawing the basic configuration, and Romano and the other apprentices, but especially Romano, would take over from there, the reason for Raphael's stupendous turn out. On Raphael's death Romano and Gianfrancesco set their sights on completing Raphael's unfinished works, which were numerous. Then Clement VII decided to build a wonderful palace, eventually known as the Villa Madama, surrounded by parks, gardens and lakes, and named Romano responsible for it all. As an accomplished architect this posed no problem and Romano was excellent at making the drawings for the paintings and frescoes that would decorate the interior, but he lacked the patience to do the work himself as a painting could take months, even years. His paintings are therefore less dynamic, less emotional than his drawings.

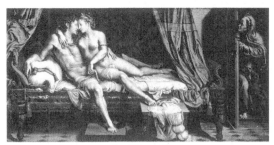

Romano's *Two Lovers*

Romano knew the Duke of Mantua Federico Gonzaga who, learning that the pope was building a new palace, wanted one too, the future Palazzo Te. How he got Clement to free Romano is not known, but he left Rome for Mantua where the duke provided him with a beautiful home with handsome boy servants as the duke too appreciated healthy lads. With his usual skill, Romano brought the palace to completion and had artists brought in to furnish the interior, all for fantastic sums that the duke had no problem paying. The palace, away from the center of Mantua, was known to be for the sexual pleasure of the duke who nonetheless up and died, giving great pain to Romano as both men had been close, sharing not only girls and boys but also the pornographic sketches for which Romano would become renown. Shortly afterwards Romano too died in Mantua, at age 54, leaving but one son who very soon joined his father in the family tomb.

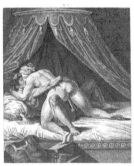

MARS ET VENUS

At times I wonder how great a writer Proust would have been had he told the true story of his life, instead of giving his male lovers and other male personages female identities. I think his work would have been a true masterpiece instead of an endless oeuvre that everyone begins but no one-- or nearly no one--finishes. The same holds true for Vasari. As I wrote in the chapter on Cellini, he loved sex with boys even to the point of injuriously scratching them in the throes of orgasm, as Cellini tells us in his autobiography. In his life of Roman, Vasari says not a world concerning the pornographic *I Modi* that he and all the literati in Italy and beyond (including Shakespeare) knew about and ardently collected.

Romano was a fun-loving man who once sponsored a dinner in honor of a boy who had been cured of syphilis. The men were invited to bring their mistresses. One of the guests was Cellini who brought his current boyfriend, age 16, dressed as a girl. When a diner introduced his hand into the lass's panties and found out the truth, the men broke up in laughter and several of the mistresses left in a huff.

Romano was the only Renaissance artist referred to by Shakespeare in his *The Winter's Tale* in which he speaks of "that rare Italian master, Giulio Romano."

The *I Modi* were 32 paintings, 16 of which represented scenes of heterosexual intercourse, 16 others of homosexual couplings. Romano drew them and the poet Aretino wrote dirty sonnets to accompany them. The first 16 were reproduced by the engraver Marcantonio Raimondi and gained such notoriety that they were banned and destroyed under the order of the pope. But they had been more or less well copied by others and exist to this day. The 16 homosexual drawings were considered too outrageous to be copied, and so have been entirely lost.

Romano was in Mantua during a visit of the Holy Roman Emperor Charles V and was responsible for the construction of the triumphal arches under which Charles passed, as well as the decorations for the feasts and joists, and the creation of the costumes and masks. Later he built gardens, chapels, houses and brought fresh water from nearby sources into Mantua to fill pools and lakes. He became wealthy and his studio was a popular shelter for apprentices, models, clients and the upper classes who stopped by to slum, to gossip and to pick up boys.

Cellini attended a party given by Giulio Romano, a painter notorious for his *I Modi* sexual-intercourse drawings. Romano thought it would be amusing to have a dinner in which the men invited their mistresses (whom Cellini reveals later as being, for the most part, whores). Cellini had none, but he did have a boy of wondrous beauty, 16, whom he dressed as a girl. "Diego had a handsome figure, and a complexion of marvelous brilliancy. The outlines of his head and face were far more beautiful than those of the antique Antinous. When I begged him to let me array him in women's clothes he readily complied." Diego is recorded to have made such a splash that one of the men present fell to his knees before him and said, "Behold ye of what sort are the angels of paradise!" One of the mistresses left in a huff, followed by another when one of the men put his hand in the little lady's panties and discovered the truth. The men broke up in laughter and Diego, the "girl" of wondrous beauty, was said to have passed an equally wondrous night. (The details of which, alas, are not found in Cellini's book.) The mistress who had left in a huff was a whore named Pantasilea who decided to get revenge against Cellini by seducing one of his boyfriends, the handsome Luigi Pulci. Both Luigi and Cellini were free to go with other boys, but Cellini did not want him to go with Pantasilea. Cellini had met Luigi when the lad was sick with syphilis and provided the best doctors for him, never leaving his bedside until he was well. He, and everyone who met Luigi, fell in love with him. He was said to have had a beautiful voice and sang in public, his beauty and talent attracting even Michelangelo who followed him assiduously from performance to performance, and became his lover. It was because Cellini had nursed the boy back to health that he now got his absolute assurance that he would not sleep with Pantasilea. She nonetheless succeeded in alluring the boy into her bed, an act that infuriated the artist no end, even though, as I said, he partook of any boy who caught his fancy--and they were numerous--no matter if they were connected to one of his friends or not--meaning that if a friend's back was turned Cellini never hesitated to steal his boy. Cellini therefore decided to waylay the couple and teach them a lesson. Several days later they had all gone to a party but Cellini left while Luigi and the whore were engaged in necking. He went to the whore's house and waited for them outside. His ire mounted when they returned, their bodies as entwined as his and Luigi's had been when they were going steady. Cellini jumped from behind the tree where he was hiding and hit Luigi with his sword, a glancing blow that also struck Pantasilea, "hitting her full on the nose and mouth," wrote Cellini. Cellini was arrested and shouted to Luigi, as he was being marched away, that if he continued seeing Pantasilea he'd break his neck. Shortly afterwards Luigi Pulci was caracoling his horse in an attempt to impress Pantasilea. It had rained and the horse slipped, falling on the boy, breaking his neck.

François I
1494 - 1547

François, who had already lost his virginity to his sister at age 10, was a lad 6 ½ feet tall and so big some girls couldn't accommodate him although most tried, and, it was said, virgins literally lined up around his bed awaiting their chance to be deflowered--his specialty. His bed, as I've mentioned but can't help repeating, even accompanied him while he was out hunting, using it between kills, to the utter amazement of Henry VIII who had accompanied the king during his visit to France (Henry went far in such things, very far even, but not *that* far). François took whomever he wanted from the nobility, whether the ladies liked it or not, and apparently not all did as one woman had her husband infect himself with syphilis before infecting her so that she could infect the king. Another woman had her face slashed, which didn't dissuade François as it wasn't her face that interested him.

François offered him a commission: six colossal gods and six goddesses, all in silver, more than life-size as François wanted them his height, the purpose of which would be to hold candlesticks. That he asked Cellini to create these giant candelabras, holding three or more candles, was a surprise, given the expense of the project, as Cellini was only noted for his belt buckles, silver plates and vases.

Cellini set to work making a clay model of one of the statues, a male figure, that was cast in bronze over which he hammered sheets of silver with a wooden hammer. During this time Cellini had problems with accountants, with jealous artists who badmouthed him and, far more deadly, with Madame d'Étampes, François' mistress, whose ass (to be honestly frank) he just hadn't sufficiently kissed.

The day came for Cellini to present the finished statue to the king and his mistress. ''The Jupiter was raising his thunderbolt with the right hand in the act of hurling it; his left hand held the globe of the world. ''Among the flames of the thunderbolt I had very cleverly introduced a torch of white wax.'' Cellini had the king observe the statue from several angles, informing him that a sculpture should always be viewed from at least eight different standpoints. Cellini had draped some tissue around the statue's private parts, knowing a woman would be present, but when d'Étampes saw the statue she suggested to the king that the tissue was there to hid some imperfection. Cellini had Ascanio take it away. Madame d'Étampes stared at the incredible detail of the pubic bush, balls, penis and ample foreskin, and Cellini asked, ''Do you find it all as it should be?'' Madame d'Étampes left the room in a huff. As soon as she was gone the king ''exploded with laughter,'' says Cellini. The statue had taken 4 years to make, at the cost of 40,000 francs.

Casanova
1725 - 1798

As stated, in ancient times men were omnisexual, taking their pleasure with what was often closest at hand. The Greek penchant was boys, but Greek males had no difficulty in producing children (16), and in Sparta the law obliged them to have children, although they did it to such a limited extent that Sparta, due to its lack of new soldiers, soon disappeared: the Spartans were quite simply ejecting their semen into male buttocks far more often than between female thighs (14). The evil influence of religion made male-male sex punishable by burning at the stake, even if, during the Renaissance, men got off lightly throughout the enlightened de' Medici years (6), when literally every man was copulating with every other man and boy. The homosexual Dark Ages that followed ended in a surge of erotic activity among Prussian men, at which time the word homosexual itself was invented by the German Karl Ulrichs in 1862 (15).

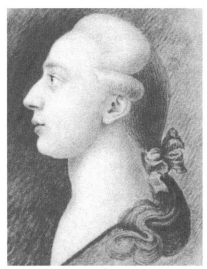

Casanova was not a beauty, but possessed endless charm.

And Casanova in all this? The best résumé of what he was doing is found in *Wikipedia*, which ranges his biographers into three categories: ''Casanova's first editor, Jean Laforgue, ruthlessly censored every reference to the autobiographer's homosexual activity. Since then critical reaction has varied widely, from John Masters who cites Casanova's limited admissions of same-sex eroticism as proof of his essential bisexuality, to J. Rives Childs who strains to divorce Casanova's sexual practice from his sexual orientation by ascribing his 'rare act of pederasty' less to inclination than curiosity, to Michel Delon who sidesteps the question of Casanova's possible homosexuality altogether, associating his behavior with traditional early modern libertinism in which a mature man's erotic attentions might be directed indiscriminately toward women or boys without compromising his sexual identity.'' Meaning that Casanova was a man clearly of his times, in no way immune to a pair of charming--most probably hairless--boy buttocks.

Serenissima homosexuality wasn't aided by religion which cast a leaden curtain over sex between males, even when such sex was *the* major outlet for priests and cardinals. Added to this is the age-old prohibition against incest, which has for its basis the evolutionary need for the survival of the species, a survival that is endangered by consanguinity and, especially, the waste of a man's seed in male-male sex and in onanism.

Ian Kelly, in his *Casanova: Actor Lover Priest Spy*, 2008, writes: ''The modern concept of bisexuality, no less than of homosexuality, didn't really exist in the 18ᵗʰ century, and the conception of sexual preference was on the whole a much more fluid affair. It seems that Casanova was a man who in sex, as in life, wanted to taste all the flavors on offer.'' Kelly goes on to suggest that if Casanova didn't go into more detail concerning his encounters with men and boys, it was ''to quash rumors afoot in Venice that his rise to prominence was courtesy of his having been the rent boy of his first patron, Meteo Giovanni Bragadin.''

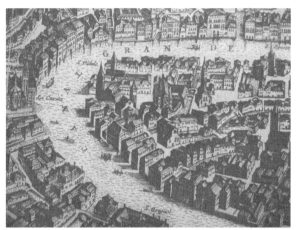

Venice at the time of Casanova.

Casanova slept with few men and women, perhaps 130 in all (compared to don Giovanni's 1,003), but his lasting influence is thanks to the erotic way in which he wrote about his conquests in his memoirs, an example being two sisters he would possess: ''two buds who only wait for a breath of love to come into bloom.'' [A boy, in any of today's dormitories, can outdo Casanova in a year, although he may have difficulty keeping up with the brilliant novelist George Simenon who had had 10,000 (girls).]

Billions of years of evolution has placed the survival of the species as the number one exigency. Here Casanova hit the nail on the head when evoking the very ''soul'' that was the foundation of his existence, ''soul'', in Casanova's case, referring to his dick. His dick was his *raison d'être*, as it is ours--*évolution oblige*. [''I live for, with and by my balls'' Errol Flynn would later proclaim (3).]

One overlooks, too, Casanova's immense literary output: He wrote 42 books and plays, he translated the *Iliad*, penned a 5-volume science-fiction novel, wrote treatises on mathematics and even opera libretti, all in addition to his 12-volumn *The Story of My Life*, a bestseller then as today, written in French, the language most used at the time.

Born in 1725 in Venice, he was stimulated sexually very early on by the daughter of the family who adopted him, although his first penetration would wait until age 17, when it took place with two sisters. He came 4 times with one, her trusting husband asleep in a room nearby, and then took her virgin 17-year-old sister, just weeks before her wedding. [Byron had been sexually manipulated by a female servant at age 9.] He had wanted to enter the clergy, but was expulsed when found in bed with a fellow seminary student. He went on to have a child, a girl he would later impregnate. At age 19 he traveled to Constantinople where he and a friend spied on a group of naked harem girls, the friend, a Turk, manipulating Casanova's aroused member through his clothing. ''It would have been impolite to refuse,'' wrote Casanova, ''I would have shown myself ungrateful.''

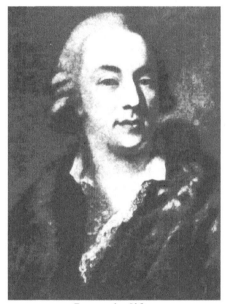

Later in life.

One of his most extraordinary conquests was of Bellino, a girl who passed as a boy, doting herself with an artificial penis. Casanova was attracted by both her feminine and masculine attributes, discovering that it was a girl only at the time of penetration, an act that would leave her with a child she later--still posing as a boy--said was her brother. Even the supposed love of his life, a certain Henrietta, had at first attracted him when he saw her disguised as a man, during her flight from a brutal husband.

At age 28 the Venetian Inquisition received word from various sources of Casanova's preference for younger and younger prey, boys often from the nobility he was tutoring. He was arrested and sent to the Leads, an escape-proof prison he miraculously escaped from. He went to the Paris of Louis XV, himself a debauched lover of orgies. It was there Casanova thought up the idea of a national lottery, which would make him rich enough to carry on his career of international seducer. His charm, his daring escape from prison, as well as the relating of other adventures, made him an indispensible guest at dinners, as would later be the case for the likes of Oscar Wilde and Truman Capote. His deep involvement in the mystical and mysterious Cabbala provided him with powers of healing and the ability to bestow eternal life, an enormous aphrodisiac to the countless-- and extremely wealthy--women he possessed, one of whom he even promised to transmigrate into the body of a male infant. One woman, a Marquess, took her pleasure in watching Casanova take the virginity of the young girls she offered him (deflowering virgins would soon become his greatest pleasure). He gambled, he screwed, and he had the inevitable duels that went along with his seducing the wives of others.

Due to depression and his syphilitic body, he decided to do away with himself, intending to jump from the Westminster Bridge, his pockets weighed down with lead shot. The year was 1763 and he was 38. A passer-by, a friend, unaware of what Casanova was planning, invited him for a meal. Restored, Casanova went on to additional exploits, one being the impregnation of his own daughter, a service he rendered her because her husband was unable to father children. She thusly had Casanova's.

He lost his looks, and his fortune through gambling, and took on work as a librarian, dying, alone, at age 73.

He never stopped imagining ''that something better was coming along'' wrote his biographer Ian Kelly, which is, I might add, the motor of us all.

Lord Byron
1788 – 1824

Byron lived in an age when men were hanged for their love of males and/or pilloried, caged in public and punched by sticks, eyes stove in and throats pierced, at times causing death. The high and mighty in England didn't necessarily escape [although most did], as shown by Oscar Wilde's trial for homosexuality, a man whose plays were immensely popular then as they are today. There was also the threat of blackmail that led to many suicides. To be hanged, both penetration and ejaculation had to be proved in a court of law, no easy affair. In France laws against sodomy were dropped after the Revolution, in 1791, and many other countries like Italy and Spain followed. But not England. Yet school was a protected sanctum, where boys could enjoy their puberty more or less unhampered. Boys were locked in their dormitories at night, left to themselves, at times exhausting their young bodies in orgies that would have impressed the Romans. *All* boarding schools were rife with sex. H. Montgomery Hyde, who later lost his seat in the House of Commons because of his plea for understanding concerning homosexuals, quoted a student, Addington Symonds: ''The talk in the dormitories and studies was of the grossest character, with repulsive scenes of onanism, mutual masturbation and obscene orgies of naked boys in bed together. There was no refinement, just animal lust.'' The first order that Thackeray received on his first day at school from a schoolmate was ''Come & frig me,'' he wrote later (8). Byron had innumerable lovers, and it is believed that his sex life began as early as age 9 when a servant aroused him sexually by taking him in her mouth. It had long been a custom in Sardinia for mothers to soothe their baby boys by taking the entirety of their sexual apparatus in their mouths, a measure said to have instantly calmed theirs sons. Later Byron claimed to have read Arabian erotica at age 10. His earliest pre-school crushes seemed to have been with girls, and girls would bring him pleasure throughout his life [pleasure for Byron's friends too, as Byron would often turn his mistresses over to them]. Had not the dangers of the pillory, hanging, blackmail and public scandal been real, he might have had far more homosexual experiences than heterosexual.

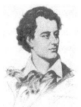

Byron

In 1808 he decided to go to the Orient. Boys he met along the way stirred him sexually and even in Falmouth he wrote to friends at Cambridge about the remarkably handsome lads, one of which he compared to Apollo's lover Hyacinth (16). He employed the word coitus throughout his letters, perhaps taking it from the *Satyricon* where Eumolpus tells how, after much trickery, he had full and complete intercourse with the boy he had been after [plenum et optabilem coitum]. He went to Albania where he found the most splendid boys he had ever seen, and then went on to Athens where he heard the story of Hadrian and Antinous (7), and where he went from boy to boy, writing home that he had had 200 couplings [''two hundred *pl and opt Cs*''], so many that he was becoming tired of them, he wrote. In Athens he visited the site of the two lovers Aristogeiton and Harmodius (16). He went on to Leuctra where the Sacred Band of lovers defeated the Spartans and then to the Thermopylae where Leonidas saved us all from Persian barbarism at the head of 150 Spartan couples formed of lovers and their beloveds. He swam in the Hellespont and went on to Troy, battlegrounds of Achilles and Patroclus (14). In a letter, he regretted that the shepherds in his day did not resemble, in beauty, Paris, the abductor of Helen.

He had to be careful in what he wrote home: In one letter he admitted to receiving ''as many kisses as would have sufficed for a boarding school.'' In another ''one boy had ambrosial curls hanging down his amiable back'' and in another place he and a boy ''traveled very much enamoured.'' In still another letter he asks the reader to tell a friend that he had finally ''had'' a Greek boy they had known at Cambridge, whom Byron looked up in his native Athens, one of the few he didn't pay for.

He returned to England where men were being hung for ''unnatural crimes,'' two per year. Prison and blackmail, as well as being ostracized by one's peers, were current. The accusation of having committed a homosexual crime would bring out a mob of hundreds into the streets, and the accused had to be protected by large numbers of police. A lieutenant was caught amusing himself with a drummer boy of 16, two years after Byron's return; both were hanged. In the crowd observing the hanging was the Duke of Cumberland, who just missed inheriting the English throne. Nine months before the hanging his valet had been found dead, killed by the duke, thought some, because the valet was blackmailing him for having sex with another of the duke's male servants--every reason for Byron to make good use of whatever heterosexual blood he had within him when seeking pleasure. That he did not exclusively do so is proof of his deep attraction to boys (8).

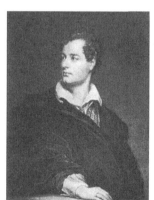

Byron, at his most beautiful.

He went to Geneva where it is said he was shunned, while in London a newspaper, the *Champion,* related that Byron was involved in a scandal but placed itself above printing the exact nature. There followed around seven years of largely heterosexual activity, including four years in Italy with a certain countess. He had met her at age 31, she 20, and her husband 54, who appealed to the pope when she left him, but because of Byron's celebrity the pope refused to intervene. Byron was happy with what the publicity was doing for his reputation as a heterosexual in Britain, but as Molière had so rightly written, *Tout le plaisir de l'amour est dans le changement*. Byron therefore decided to return to Greece, and to boys.

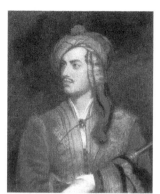

Byron in Albanian splendor.

There he met the Chalandrutsanos family, consisting of a mother who had fallen on bad times, her three daughters and Lukas, her 15-year-old son who was busy fighting the Turks for Greek independence. Youths from all over Europe, Germany, France, Spain and Italy were flocking to Greece to help the Greeks win their freedom, but due to Greek incompetence, whose who survived returned in rags. Byron took Lukas in hand and wherever they went Byron was well received, thanks to his reputation and wealth. He provided the boy with a uniform and pistols, and welcomed him into his entourage as a page, the usual cover for rent boys. He had Lukas read ancient Greek texts, certainly those tainted with Greek love, and like any boy Lukas' age, and having lived under the Turks, the boy certainly recognized the intentions behind Byron's largesse.

Even at age 23 Byron had envisioned suicide, but at that age he was sexually fulfilled, and so such thoughts meant little in comparison to now, nearly 36, his hair thinning, his teeth bad and his body fat. He was far from sexually satiated now, so thoughts of suicide, on the battlefield, alongside his Lukas, were attractive. The revenge of age is total. Byron's reputation and money could buy him consolation, but the mirror was there to remind him of the inevitable ravages of time. Lucky were those like Achilles, like Patroclus, Alexander and Hephaestion, who left early, in possession of their physical force and beauty.

Lukas was perhaps there to consol him because he shared Byron's bed, as related by numerous sources. But Lukas appeared unhappy, and

Byron's gifts to him, gilded pistols, gold-laced jackets and a beautiful saddle, seemed to have done little to lessen what appeared to have been the boy's disdain for Byron. Perhaps the boy in no way shared Byron's bent, perhaps he would have preferred someone younger with a beautiful body. A man throwing himself at a disdainful boy is sad, especially for a boy who had known the luxury of love and fulfilled desire since his early puberty, as had Byron.

Byron wrote poems to the boy, so sexually discreet that it's difficult to know what he's talking about, yet in the reality of his daily life he was telling friends that his ''cock still has spring in it''.

This may have been so, but there was daily less spring in his health. He suffered from fevers, perhaps the malaria he had contracted in the South of France as a boy, and syphilis. He had dizzy spells and weakness. Bloodletting, still popular, in no way helped, and some say it even killed him. In 1824 he was carried away by fever, certainly not to a better place since it's difficult to imagine a destiny as fulfilling in love, in art, in sexual bliss as that having been lived by Byron. He died at 36, the exact age of his father. A few months later, victim of the Greek War for Independence, Lukas followed. [The full life of Byron can be found in my book *Christ Has His John, I Have My George: The History of British Homosexuality*.]

Rudolph Valentino
1895 - 1926

One of Alla's first most notable visitors was Valentino, from around 1924 to his death in 1926. He rode over horseback from the Paramount studio lot, and during one luncheon he met Alla's set designer, Winifred Shaughnessy, who was also Alla's lover. When Valentino decided he needed a wife for publicity reasons he chose Shaughnessy, which greatly angered Alla but opened up a whole new life of wealth for Winifred who changed her name to Natcha Rambova, and it was as such that she tried out for roles in films, landing a part in *When Love Grows Cold*. She eventually calmed Alla by frequently attending her lesbian sewing circles. Alla had also previously introduced Valentino to his first wife, who returned to live on the Garden grounds with Alla after her divorce from Valentino.

The marriage between Valentino and Rambova was highly dysfunctional. Born to Mormons in Salt Lake City, Utah, Rambova's mother, thanks to several fructuous marriages, saw to it that her daughter was educated in Britain and that she took ballet lessons in New York. One of the young girl's first lovers worked as a designer for DeMille and she followed him to Hollywood to become, herself, a costume designer. Although she shared Spiritualism with Valentino, and later wrote she would treasure her honeymoon with him all her life [Valentino had often said he was an ace at handling his 10 inches, and could bring pleasure to whomever he ''honored''], she nevertheless wanted to continue her career, her major disagreement with Valentino who wanted a son and wanted her home to care for Valentino himself. His Italian male chauvinism eventually abandoned him to the extent that it was she who ruled the roost, deciding even the roles in films he would accept to play. Her influence was so disruptive that only when she was banned from the studios did Valentino find work again. After Valentino's death she remarried, founded a dress shop on Fifth Avenue, N.Y., taught Spiritualism and Egyptology, passing away at age 66 from heart failure, remembered from then on as Valentino's second wife, Mrs. Valentino.

Rodolfo Alfonso Raffaello Pierre Filibert Guglielmi di Valentina d'Antonguolla, ''Valentino'', was born in 1895. He didn't start off with a life as incredibly adventurous as Errol Flynn's or David Niven's, but he was rough and undisciplined, sent from school to school for being uncontrollable. At first he chose agriculture as his life's work and went to school in Genoa where at 5' 11'' he took up weight-lifting and football. His father had left him money he used to travel to Paris where he went to clubs like the Alcazar and picked up the Apache, a wild dance in which the barely dressed girl was hoisted about, flung like a ragdoll, slapping the male while he threatened her with a knife, she a prostitute, he her pimp. Getting a hard-on with a man showing him the movements, the man loaned Valentino his wife to straighten the boy out, but in the end Valentino got the man.

He found work at Maxim's as a dancer, paid by women per dance. As they were rich, and as he later stated that fucking had always come easily to him, he made good money. He specialized in the tango and had his trousers tailored so as to show his muscular buttocks and extensive manhood. Soon named the Italian Stallion, he thrilled the ladies, who requested private dance lessons. His reputation was augmented when it became known that he was too much of a mouthful for most of them, but just right for a pussy needing stretching.

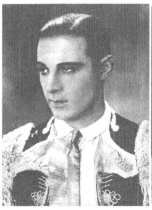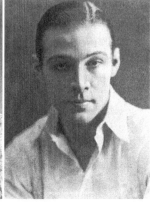

One of Valentino's rich clients was a woman who shot her husband dead, and Rudy, afraid of being dragged into the trial, fled to California. In Los Angeles he hooked up with an actor who convinced him to try out for work as a studio extra.

He became a member of the Torch Club, at around $1,000 a month, that had a special room, # 23, above which was a two-way mirror. New boys were given the room where they fucked in full view of a hidden audience, jacking off. The first boy he went into the room with was Richard Barthelmess, both unaware of the voyeurs. Richard later posed nude for friends and was said to have been huge. Rudy met producers at the club and got numerous small roles. He was soon servicing actresses for money, several a day, and still had enough for Richard whom he continued to see.

Valentino got the chief role in *The Four Horsemen of the Apocalypse* during which Novarro, a bit-player, told him that Valentino was the love of his life. In thanks Valentino gave Novarro a 10" bronze sculpture of his phallus, the one Novarro purportedly choked to death on at the end of his kidnapping/murder, whose story will be told later. During a party Valentino and his girlfriend were introduced as Snow White and Mr. 7 Inches, so the exact size of his manhood is unknown.

The success of *The Four Horsemen of the Apocalypse* rocketed him to fame, but he was so imbued with himself that he made increasing demands for more money, causing bad blood among directors and costing him good roles, some of which went to Novarro. He left Metro for Famous Players where his contract went from $350 a week to $750, this during the depression when one earned a dollar a day, if lucky.

His film *The Sheik* was taken from an English book found nearly pornographic, about a woman kidnapped by an Arab who used her for his sexual pleasure in his tent, telling her that she had it better with him than his men, and then the shocking discloser that she ended up liking "it". The amusing aspect is that the female lead gave interviews comparing Latin lovers to Americans, although in reality she preferred women and was thought to have been a virgin [to men at least].

His fan mail exploded, with women requesting pubic hair clippings and men underwear he ejaculated in--in return for money. He married. Divorced. And immediately married again, so rapidly that the first marriage hadn't come through and he was indicted for bigamy. He got out of it when his new wife declared their marriage had not been consummated, and was thusly null and void.

His next film was the one he preferred, *Blood and Sand*, he as a matador. He was 26 and apparently loved to wear the matador costume from then on as a preliminary to sex.

In the film *Young Rajah* Valentino played a student who, in one scene where the rowers were wearing shorts and carrying a boat over their heads, was bawled out by the director who thought he was sporting a boner as a prank, and ordered him to take a cold shower. Valentino lowered the shorts to prove that he was in his normal flaccid state.

Valentino was said to have had such magnetism that even homophobes wanted to have sex with him, wrote Jacques Hébertot, whose pleasure was touring French streets to pick up boys that he turned into actors. Hébertot's greatest discovery was Gérard Philipe, one of France's truly great and beloved artists. Hébertot introduced Valentino to André Daven that Hébertot said was the world's most beautiful boy. Stuck on himself, Daven told the great Valentino that if he wanted him he'd have to give him a role in one of his films. Valentino replied that he'd give the boy a role in *all* his films, an anecdote revealed by David Bret in his *Valentino*, a wonderful biography.

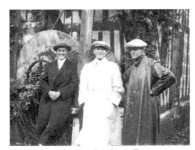

Valentino in the middle, Daven on the right
[sorry, it's the best photo I can find].

In 1923, at age 28, Valentino signed a contract with United Artists that paid $10,000 a week and 42% of United Artists' profits, plus a bungalow, a maid, a dresser and a chef. The only provision was that his wife, the harridan Rambova, have no say whatsoever concerning the films and the filming of the films. He signed, especially as Daven was still at his side. [After Valentino's death Daven returned to Paris and to Hébertot, and then literally disappeared from the face of the planet.]

Valentino bought a boat, packed with boys, usually nude, and went to Catalina Island. The fun and games continued at his home, Falcon Lair, where Valentino especially liked to screw on the roof of his car. Valentino declared a ''no fuck Friday'', Bret tells us, reserved for outings to things like boxing matches. But as soon as midnight struck, it was back home and orgy time.

It was around then that he began suffering from abdominal pains.

He went to Paris where he fell for a ballet choreographer who chose his boy-for-the-night by lining up lads [mostly his dancers] in a row and measuring their dicks hard. Valentino took part and won for that night. One boy called his endowment Herculean.

His doctors were certain they could successfully operate and cure his abdominal stress. They couldn't. At 31 he was dead. The end of a near-perfect life.

Porfirio Rubirosa

Porfirio Rubirosa Ariza, 1909-1965, was an international jetsetter playboy, known for his sexual prowess with women, two of whom, his wives, were the richest in the world. He was also said to have been Dominican dictator Rafael Trujillo's hit man, assassinating political opposition to the regime. He was a polo player and race car driver, and it was at the wheel of his Ferrari that he crashed into a tree in the Bois de Bologna, killing himself at age 56 [the perfect death because it was rapid and unexpected].

Howard Hughes
1905 - 1975

Howard Hughes had had them all, but his friendship with Cary Grant lasted the longest, half a century. In Darwin Porter's *Howard Hughes Hell's Angel* we learn of a cruise on Hughes's *Southern Cross* where a friend reported: ''It appeared they were on their honeymoon ... lying nude on the deck with their arms around each other.... Neither of them seemed to care what the all-male crew thought. I couldn't help notice that Hughes's endowment looked two and a half times bigger than that of Cary's.'' Porter relates: ''When Hughes learned he had syphilis, he called Cary Grant and told him. Since he'd had sex with Cary only recently, he feared that the actor might also have contracted the disease.'' At the end of his life Hughes told Grant that he had been his only loyal friend, that women had just wanted roles in movies and boys hundred-dollar bills. Howard Hughes was bisexual, whose father's wealth and his own curiosity led to early sexual discovery. At age 13 he visited Hollywood where a bisexual man and wife awoke him to every erogenous zone on his body--zones responsible for sexual arousal and orgasm. Years later, actor Jack Buetel complained that Howard Hughes would continually bring him to orgasm in order to lap up his virility, which would reinforce, Howard believed, his own, at the same time making sure that Buetel got good roles.

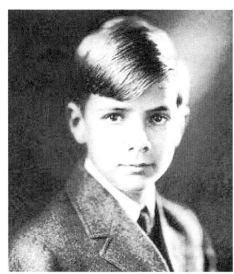

Howard Hughes at the age when a bisexual man and wife awoke every erogenous zone on his body.

Darwin Porter, in his *Howard Hughes Hell's Angel*, writes that during Hughes's first night with Power he had expected someone aggressive. What he got was a bottom "who wanted to be deeply penetrated. Again and again", while whispering "flattery into the ear of his top." When Tyrone learned that Hughes had had Errol Flynn he begged him for an introduction. Hughes invited Flynn and Tyrone on his yacht the *Southern Cross* along with a Navy man known to be well endowed. The Navy man serviced all three, stating later that both Hughes and Flynn were "sword swallowers", while Tyrone preferred passive sodomy. Hughes was into voyeurism, the Navy man claimed, and jerked off while watching Flynn giving it to Tyrone. Tyrone Power was so good-looking that his boss Darryl Zanuck said, "The handsome bastard gave me a hard-on when we were in the sauna together, and I'm the only real bonafide heterosexual in all of Hollywood."

Tyrone invited Hughes to Mexico for the filming of *Blood and Sand*. Hughes told a friend that sex was still good with Tyrone, and "he's the only man who can reach climaxes while you're chomping down on his nipples." During the production of *Captain from Castile* Hughes--in Acapulco with Lana Turner and Power--screwed Tyrone while Tyrone screwed Lana. "It was one of the best orgasms I've ever had," Hughes later said.

Darwin Porter in his *Howard Hughes Hell's Angel* claims that Cooper was going with Rod La Rocque who had been intimate with Hughes. When Hughes demonstrated interest in the young Cooper, Rocque said, "Go for it ... he'll drop his pants for anybody, male or female, who he thinks is loaded.'' Hughes was said to have been Gary's sugar daddy during his first years in Hollywood.

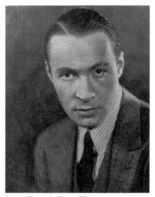

Rod La Rocque

It is impossible to know the real cause of Clark Gable's homophobia. As soon to be reported, Gable had given himself to William Haines in order to procure a role, and the more Haines declined in preeminence and the more Gable rose in public esteem--to the point that Judy Garland composed a song in his honor in *Broadway Melody*, unique in cinema history--the more Haines told one and all how he had had Gable pinned up against a wall while Haines pounded him from behind. Haines told Howard Hughes that Gable would drop his trousers for either sex, if it would lead to a film contract, something Hughes himself tried. Others suggested that Gable had been a hustler during his youth, all of which may have combined to make Gable hypersensitive about his sexuality. During the filming of *Gone with the Wind* Gable, now King of Hollywood, got homosexual George Cukor fired when the director jokingly questioned him on the pervasive rumors concerning both Howard Hughes and William Haines, and throughout the filming Gable never ceased to show his disdain for Leslie Howard, a homosexual and a regular at the Garden of Allah thanks to the appeal of its British residents. Howard detested his role in *Gone with the Wind*, writing, ''I hate the damn part. I'm not nearly beautiful or young enough for Ashley, and it makes me sick being fixed up to look attractive.'' In the *film* he was 21, in *reality* 46.

Hughes tried to get Gable in the sack and arranged a luncheon. The conversation, records Darwin Porter, was all pussy, Gable stating that he went for anything from hash slingers to call girls, ''All pussies are dark at night. Love 'em and leave 'em.'' Because Haines had told Hughes that Gable would allow himself to be taken in order to get a role, Hughes told Clark that he was a natural for the role Gable was dying for, Hildy Johnson in *The Front Page*. Hughes invited Gable to fly with him to San Francisco, and when he returned to Hollywood Haines asked him what had taken place, but Hughes remained uncharacteristically silent. Some thought something *had* taken place, but that Howard had been unhappy with the result, perhaps because Clark had a small dick [confirmed by girls he bedded], perhaps because he was known to come to quickly, but perhaps also because he had a reputation for not being clean down there. At any rate, during the filming of *Gone with the Wind* director George Cukor kidded Gable about what had taken place between him and Hughes and Haines. The homophobe Gable gave the homosexual Cukor the dirtiest look he was capable of, and never spoke to him again--which was not for long because Cukor was soon removed. By the way, Hughes made sure that Gable didn't get the role of Hildy Johnson, stating that his ears were too big. As far as we know, Gable's only homosexual *faux pas* was with actor Billy Haines.

Durex research states that the average number of sexual relations is 127 a year. Men under 30 are said to be able to copulate 4 times a night, over 30 around twice a week. This of course varies hugely. As written, Warren Beatty has had over 12,000 and a certain lap dancer claimed that Ronaldinho had her 8 times in one evening. Mae West had an incalculable number of males, as did Tullulah Bankhead, Joan Crawford and Lana Turner who loved hers big, as with her lover Johnny Stompanato. Take this extract from my book *Cesare Borgia*: ''When the time came, Cesare set off for France with cartloads of precious gifts. He was beautifully dressed in black and white velvet, pearls and gold chains and precious gems attached to his clothes and boots, his horse was attired in gorgeous livery and silver bells. He was accompanied by dozens of mules covered in satin, in cloth of gold, dozens of grooms in crimson velvet, noblemen in gold and silver, musicians, playing trumpets, all of which made the French laugh at his pomposity. He knelt to kiss Louis's foot but was halted and allowed the king's hand instead. In addition to the wealthy display, Cesare had not forgotten the cardinal's hat to be presented to Georges d'Amboise, Louis's trusted counselor. Cesare was offered the sister of the King of Navarre, sixteen-year-old Carlotta. Alexander was hoping for a better match for his son, a girl from the king's own family, but allowed the marriage because Cesare seemed happy with her, and Alexander even gave the girl's brother, Amanieu d'Albret, a cardinal's hat. Louis wrote Alexander a description of the wedding night, telling the pope that Cesare honored his wife eight times in a row. Louis added that he had done the same with his new wife--thanks to the divorce Alexander had accorded him--but confessed that he had nonetheless done less well as his sessions had been broken up, twice before dinner, six times afterwards. Alexander replied that he was awed by the king and proud of his son but not surprised by his virility. Carlotta was immediately pregnant with a girl, Cesare's only known child.''

Homosexuals cannot only have sex 8 times a night, but they can easily do so with 8 different boys. College students, today, can also pulverize the records of vintage cocksmen.

SEX AND ATHLETES

Athletes are convinced that sex before a competition ''weakens legs'', and Plato, in 444 B.C., wrote that ''competitors before races should avoid sexual intimacy.'' Mohammad Ali abstained from sex seven weeks before a match, and an Olympic runner stated that ''Sex makes me happy. Happy people do not run a 3:47 mile.''

The key to whether sex weakens a boy's performance in sports seems to be *when* he has sex. A study in 1995 measured two men on a treadmill, one who had had sex twelve hours earlier, but not the second. There was no difference in performance. Yet some trainers refer to another study, in 1968, that showed that men who had not had sex for six days did better than those who did so the night before.

Follow-up studies indicate that having sex several hours before a competition has no effect, while sex two hours earlier does, which begs the question because few athletes are messing around in that way just before a game. Another lad declared, ''I don't want to be distracted before any completion. Sexual encounters require effort and focus, and I want to have a clear head for a competition.'' Sexologist Jess O'Reily states that sex is the scapegoat when booze and partying are the culprits. ''It isn't sex that ruins these guys, it's staying up all night looking for it.''

After sex the hormone prolactin is freed, which induces sleep and a feeling of well-being, physical and emotional satisfaction, all of which might adversely effect an athlete's motivation and drive.

In 2000 Ian Shrier, a sports medicine specialist, stated that aggression is needed in some sports, like boxing and football, and that abstinence boosts testosterone levels that make a competitor more aggressive the longer he abstains. Another observer stated that after three months without sex testosterone levels dramatically drop to that of children, hardly conducive to aggression.

Sex therapist Eric Garrison states that it's all superstition, and that athletes tell him they don't want to jinx anything by breaking the pre-game dry spell, no matter how horny. He goes on to say that some of the best professional football, basketball and baseball athletes he'd worked with all wanted permission to have sex before or on the day of a competition, and his advice to them was to go ahead and masturbate or have consensual protected sex. Physical therapist Kosta Kokolis stated that sex before matches was beneficial because it increased blood circulation, improved mood and decreased nervousness. A college player said that "sex before a game helped relax and gave confidence. It gives you an edge."

Joe Namath told *Playboy* that the night before a game he prepared himself physically and mentally, and if that meant having a girl, he did. "If some players don't feel that way, they shouldn't."

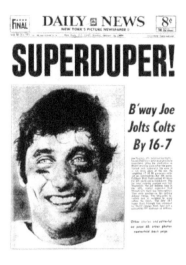

Namath

Pliny the Elder wrote, around 60 A.D., "Athletes when sluggish are revitalized by lovemaking."

The bottom line? Who really knows? [Although Namath does seem to hit the nail on the head.]

PROMESCUITY AND SEXUAL SATISFACTION

For gay men, the number of sexual partners in a male heterosexual's life is shockingly low [the reason why some homosexuals claim they are more virile than straights]. A 1994 study in the U.S. found that 20% of heterosexual men had 1 partner throughout their lives, 55% had from 2 to 20, and 25% more than 20. These numbers cover a *lifetime*, while a gay man can easily have 20 different partners in a single month of his life.

Warren Beatty's 12,000 before his marriage is far behind Castro's claim of 35,000, or Wilt Chamberland's 20,000, as stated in his autobiography. Magic Johnson said he'd had thousands, including after-game quickies in the locker room before returning to the court for postgame interviews. Charlie Sheen says he's had 5,000 and Jack Nicholson put his at 2,000. [Tennessee Williams was a genius who used his position as a Shakespeare-quality playwright to seduce boys, of whom one of the most talented was the gorgeous Warren Beatty himself, who wanted the principle role in Williams' *Roman Spring of Mrs. Stone*. Beatty and Williams were in the same hotel and Beatty showed up at his door in only a bathrobe. ''You don't have to do that,'' said Tennessee when he opened the door. Both knew he did.]

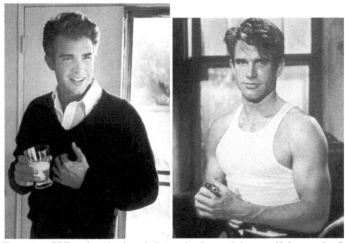

Beatty: Who in their right mind could possibly resist?

A 2014 Durex study stated that satisfaction in sex came through mutual love, freedom from stress, ability to have an orgasm, no sexual dysfunctions and frequent sex accompanied with foreplay.

The Swiss come in first in sexual satisfaction, but I personally wonder if the Swiss *think* they're satisfied because they don't know what really great sex entails. Spain comes in second, which is easy to believe, as is Italy that came in 3rd. Spaniards are rated best male lovers, although I'd put my money on Italian males, who do come in first in some studies. 90% of Spanish men and women claim to be sexually satisfied, an unbeatable number. 64% of Italian men and women claimed satisfaction, but perhaps they're just more demanding than the Spanish, and in reality they have it super good: the climate and the beauty of Italian men and women give them more potentiality for bliss than most other people in the world.

Brazilians come in 4th, and both Brazialian sexes lose their burdensome virginity earlier than in almost any other nation [*very* easy to believe].

MEAN AGE AT FIRST SEX (years)

Country	Age	Country	Age
Brazil	17.3	Ireland	18.7
Colombia	17.4	Mexico	19.1
Austria	17.5	Romania	19.3
New Zealand	17.5	Italy	19.4
Czech Republic	17.6	Poland	19.4
Germany	17.8	South Africa	19.4
Russia	17.9	Spain	19.5
Austria	18.1	Thailand	20.2
UK	18.3	Japan	20.4
Greece	18.4	Nigeria	20.6
Hungary	18.4	Hong Kong	20.8
Portugal	18.4	China	21.2
USA	18.4	Turkey	21.3
Canada	18.5	Taiwan	21.9
Croatia	18.5	Singapore	22
Netherlands	18.5	South Korea	22.1
Switzerland	18.6	India	22.5
France	18.7	Indonesia	23.6
		Malaysia	23.7

Loss of virginity by age, a Durex study result for 2012. Another study put the global average of first-time sex at 17.3 years, but the trend is definitely towards earlier sex, with 16.3 years, according to still another recent study [while here in France nearly every boy I personally know lost his cherry from the second half of age 15 to the first half of age 16.]

Brazil's 17.3 age is an average, meaning that probably lots of girls lose their virginity much younger. 82% of Brazilians have sex at least once a week, while another study has them going at it 145 times a year on the average. The climate and mixed blood, which give men huge appendages, is an assurance of sexual satisfaction.

The Greeks do it 164 times a year on the average, although only 51% state that they're fully satisfied. In general Greek men possess nice-sized weapons, and the climate encourages nudity. That and the influx of tourists are an ideal combination to content Greek males. [Another study has Greece coming in first, but with an average of 138 times a year, above what the study said was the global average of 103, with Croatia and Serbia coming in a close second and third with 134 and 128 times a year.]

Holland comes in 6th and no people has fewer hang-ups and is more willing than the Dutch. 64% say they're happy with their sex life, against 48% in the U.S. Thanks to sexual instruction in school, teen birth rate is 5.3 per 1,000, compared to 39.1 per 1,000 in the States. The world's finest homosexual saunas are in Holland, and the sex industry in general is flourishing (4).

Mexico is 7th, but the sexual exploitation of children is scandalous. India is 8th, where girls lose their virginity at age 22, nearly the longest wait in the world. Indians think Tantric sex, a great deal of time spent in foreplay, yet only 61% claim they are sexually satisfied.

Australia is 9th, where car sex seems to be popular, as well as threesomes. Aussie men have 25 different sexual partners in their lifetimes, against 13 for Americans, while Australian women have 10 different men, against 9 for American women in a lifetime.

As seen in my book *Prussian Homosexuality*, Germany invented the terms homosexual and heterosexual, and was *the* place to go for homosexual sex before W.W. II. It was the home of the first sex research centers, and today its sex education classes are top. German boys in general are beautifully hung (15).

APHRODISIACS

An aphrodisiac is any substance that increases the libido, the king of which is testosterone. I devoted a number of pages earlier to Aphrodite, the reason being her role in the lives of Hermes, Eros, Dionysus, Priapus and, now, the substances named for her and her control of the senses. I've already disclosed the use of goat gonads in Rome as aphrodisiacs, and their role as an aphrodisiac in the surgeries performed by John Brinkley. A Harvard professor, mentioned earlier, injected himself with a substance made from dog testes, and did feel a renewed vigor, probably more imagined than real; as was the life, also introduced earlier, of the man massaged by a woman using oils, while telling him how much she wanted to ride his huge dick, *his* renewed vigor was probably more real than imagined.

Agents supposed to raise testosterone levels are numerous, but the reader will have to do his own research as to their value: Wellbutrin [bupropion], bremelanotide [PT-141], melanotan II, crocin, phenethylamines [PEA], amphetamine, methamphetamine and pramipexole. Sexual arousal has also been noted in the drugs dicycloverine, hyoscyamine and scopolamine.

Here are several aphrodisiacs suggested by most health magazines: bananas; chocolate; oysters [a friend complained that he ate ten, but in bed later only six worked]; asparagus, chillies, watermelon, celery and pomegranate.

Most studies state that the above serve no purpose whatsoever as aphrodisiacs, but some--bananas and pomegranates, for example--are extremely recommended for one's general health.

Three popular aphrodisiacs:

Ginkgo biloba is a Chinese medicine that treats depression and sexual dysfunction, and appears to be a viable aphrodisiac. It has been found to stimulate attention, memory, judgment, reasoning, problem solving, decision-making and knowledge, *but only in people having difficulty in these areas*. It's been used in the treatment of dementia and Alzheimer's but with mixed results. A study has it effective in enhancing desire, erection, orgasm and ''afterglow'' [resolution].

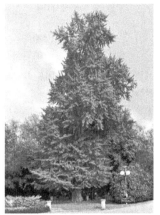

Ginkgo biloba

Ginseng has been studied and found very effective in getting a good erection. It is sold in 35 countries with sales exceeding $2 billion. Called the ''king of herbs'' it has been used since 3000 B.C.. It increases stamina, decreases fatigue and boosts the libido.

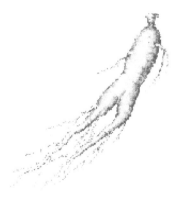

Ginseng

Maca, [*lepidium meyenii*], is a root vegetable native to the Peruvian Andes. It supposedly helps men get hard. It's called the Peruvian ginseng, and also is said to increase strength, energy and stamina, as well as the libido.

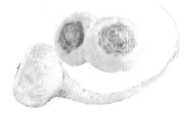

Maca

As stated, an aphrodisiac is any food or drug that causes arousal and increases pleasure and performance during sex. Before taking them a man can start out by avoiding the causes of sexual dysfunction, high blood pressure, cholesterol, diabetes and smoking, among them.

Research in the following seems to be very promising, but I can do no more than make a list that the reader can use as a basis for his own investigation. Some of the following have already been mentioned above, but are repeated because they appear in studies other than those already cited:

Chlorophytum borivilianum [CB]
Mondia whitei
Tribulus terrestris
Safron [crocus sativus]
Date palm [Phoenix dactylifera]
Eurycoma longifolia [tongkat ali or pasak bumi]
Satureja khuzestanica
Panax ginseng
Montanoa tomentosa
Terminalia catappa
Casimiroa edulis
Turnera diffusa
Pausinystalia yahimbe, dubbed the herbal Viagra by the February 1999 edition of *Environmental Nutrition in Europe*.

Rhinoceros horn and Spanish fly [cantharidan from blister beetles] are still considered aphrodisiacs by some.

Fertility saints exist, objects of reverence by girls and women who seek fruitfulness:

Saint Guerlichon at Bourge-Dieu originated as a statue of Priapus in Roman times and was so popular in restoring fertility to women that later priests transformed the statue into that of a saint. Whole pilgrimages of women flocked to the church to scrape away some of the statue's phallus that they used in the preparation of a drink. Monks were kept busy replacing the phalluses until the expense was such that they placed an apron over the instrument and told the women that their sterility would be cured by their simply lifting the apron and contemplating the saint's pud.

Saint Guénolé apparently won his reputation as a priapic patron of fertility due to the word *gignere* from the French *engendrer*, meaning to beget. His feet are pierced with needles by girls in search of a mate.

And a saint of importance to men: Saint Foutin was perhaps the first bishop of the French city of Lyon. He became an object of sexual importance because his name resembles the Old French verb *foutre*, meaning to f*ck. Today the word is slang for jizz and is used in expressions like *Va te faire foutre*, go f*ck yourself. Men came to his shrine with wax models of their impotent penises, in the hope of restored vigor. Women present were said to have been highly disturbed by the flaccid wax rods.

I'll end this chapter with the story of Victor Noir, 1848-1870, who was a French journalist. His newspaper was accused of slandering the name of Napoleon by Napoleon's great-nephew Prince Pierre Bonaparte. Bonaparte demanded that the editor of Noir's paper meet him in a duel, and Noir was sent to the prince's palace to arrange it. Inside, the prince insulted the editor, and when Noir tried to defend his boss the prince simply pulled a gun and shot him dead. Later the prince said that Noir had tried to kill him first, and that he had only defended himself. Naturally, the prince got off scot-free.

The French were on Noir's side and 100,000 accompanied him to his last resting place at the Père Lachaise Cemetery. A life-size statue of Victor Noir was sculpted by Jules Dalou, showing the outline of Noir's highly virile member. From then on the tomb was visited by so many women--who straddled it and kissed its lips--that both groin and mouth have retained their original luster.

In 2004 a fence was raised around it, but so great was the outcry from Parisian females that it was torn down. [The grave was also popular as a place of homosexual debauch.]

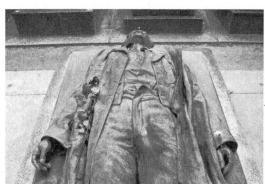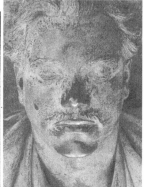

Thousands of women have ridden his manhood and kissed his lips *and feet* [sorry for the extremely poor quality of the pictures].

ALFRED KINSEY

Alfred Kinsey is an icon, one whose private life is strange nearly beyond words. Nothing has as yet replaced his sixty-year-old study, and no man has demonstrated his sexual curiosity, so outlandish that he would study the couples he hired to perform sex acts, his nose barely inches from the act itself, missing not a single odor nor sound. He loved to show off in the nude and he never hesitated to corner a fellow researcher, grope him [for Kinsey was basically homosexual], in the hope that the salary Kinsey was paying would convince him to roll over. He told his university students they were free to seek his advice on sexual matters, with the expectation that they would become hot-and-bothered enough then--or later when invited on one of his many camping expeditions--to enter into his favorite sexual pastime, mutual masturbation.

As a young man Alfred Kinsey had it all: Eagle Scout, straight-A student, high-school valedictorian, mature beyond his years, president of his class, of his Biology Club and of his Debate Team, a man they called the Second Darwin, gorgeous in high school, handsome throughout college and, later, Harvard.

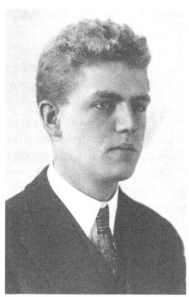

Kinsey always looked more mature than his age.

Lots of high school boys then, around 1912, didn't date, through shyness and slow maturing, while today junior high lads have sex, proof that Kinsey's famous Report, 60 years later, is completely passé. But not Kinsey's life. Photos of Kinsey show him dressed in a suit, as were the other students, a boy who took serious part in the YMCA and Boy Scouts, organizations that were Christian in character, instructing boys against sexual intercourse and masturbation: ''In the body of every boy who has reached his teens, the Creator of the universe has sown a very important fluid. This fluid is the most wonderful material in all the physical world. Some parts of it find their way into the blood, and through the blood give tone to the muscles, power to the brain, and strength to the nerves. His chest depends, his shoulders broaden, his voice changes, his ideals are enlarged. It gives him the capacity for deep feeling, for rich emotion. Pity the boy, therefore, who has wrong ideas of this important function, because they will lower his ideals of life. These organs actually secrete into the blood material that makes a boy manly, strong, and noble. Any habit which a boy has that causes this fluid to be discharged from the body tends to weaken his strength, to make him less able to resist disease.'' [From *Boy Scouts of America: The Official Handbook for Boys*, 1914, brought to us thanks to James Jones in his excellent *Alfred C. Kinsey, a life*, 1997.]

Kinsey prayed to God to release him from the terrible vice, that and his homosexuality which, in 1950, was a felony [sodomy and fellatio] in all but two states.

Most boys rationalize their masturbation because, of course, they can't stop themselves from doing it. Lots of other boys, especially in the camps

Kinsey was part of, turned masturbation into circle-jerk art, not only jerking off with friends but giving a hand to the person seated to his right. Unlike them, Kinsey felt he had to punish himself, and he did so by pushing an object, at times a straw, down the urethra of his penis and then masturbate. The pain was his punishment, pain that could last for days afterwards.

It was in college, in 1915, that Kinsey apparently admitted to himself that he was homosexual, which manifested itself in his showering and swimming with boys, naked, and fed his voyeurism in the other sports he went out for, especially tennis and golf locker rooms, because Kinsey was an athlete--as well as an accomplished pianist.

He finished college *magna cum laude* and went off to do graduate work at Harvard, in entomology. He received his doctor of science degree from Harvard around 1919 and won the Sheldon Traveling Fellowship of $1,500 [$21,000 today!], thanks to which he traveled through 36 states, 2,500 miles of which was on foot, collecting bugs. He was then taken on as an assistant professor in the Department of Zoology at Indian University in 1920, at age 26.

There, he met the girl he would eventually marry, a near societal obligation in Victorian England, when nearly all homosexuals married (8), one that existed in America too among men who refused to submit to their real sexual preference, men who were sexually confused, men who wanted to be politicians who would never be elected if the truth were known, actors who needed to save their female fans in order to keep on acting. The pattern was the same: because men didn't seek contact with women it was they who took the lead, imagining that the boy was simply shy, and often after years of basically platonic engagement, they tied the knot. With Kinsey too it was hugs and kisses, and at the time it simply didn't occur to a girl that her beau was a perverted introvert, the lesser of the terms applied to homosexuals--then as now.

Thanks to his girl Kinsey had someone who filled his solitude, who admired him, and who respected his being the perfect gentleman [while in secret he was most probably having "dirty" sex in restrooms and the bushes of parks, or, at the very least, pushing objects up his penis while he had orgasms of semen and blood], and then there was always the possibility that she would cure him of his problem [doctors persuaded actor Antony Perkins, who let *anybody* have him anally, to marry (a boyish girl had been recommended), and Perkins did finish by producing two children].

The marriage took place in 1921. He later told a friend that no sex had taken place during the honeymoon. He took control over every aspect of his wife's life, and as a university biology teacher his students found him to be arrogant, stubborn, "never giving in for any reason". He fully believed that science could free young minds and wanted his students to be free thinkers, not easy to realize, in reality, when he himself was an unmovable despotic object.

In general he supported marriage as the best way to perpetuate the species and care for the young. The place of his own wife was home caring for him--there was no question of her having a career. He treated her a hair better than the Greeks treated their wives, whose purpose was the care of the home and childrearing, all of which was incredibly strange for the man responsible for two of the world's most gigantically important books. The Kinseys soon had two children, a boy and a girl, the boy tragically dead at age three. Two other children followed, although Kinsey was said to have not been an affectionate father.

Kinsey practiced nudity at home as a way of sex education, and would pull out his member, without pretext, in front of his fellow researchers, a harbinger of later rock stars. He vacationed in nudist camps and participated in orgies, which he revealed in letters to young friends, all men. Masturbation was very often on his mind, and in conversations with male friends he always found a way to bring up the subject, and question them on how and how often they went about doing it. It was not necessarily about research, but a way of finding out if the person would be open to some mutual eroticism. The men who related this, later, had always declined, but how many had agreed, and then kept quiet? He went on field trips, staying in tents, and would spend hours telling the boys around the campfires stories about having sex, the end result was to get them hot enough so that one or several would retire to the discretion behind the canvas flaps. He also spent time in Mexico, where he would warm-up Mexican boys by telling them stories about what he had done with "hairless" girls, presumably pre-puberty, all of which put the lads in the mood to ejaculate. His vocabulary was said to have become filthy; verbally and sexually there were no limits. He left word around the campus that if students had questions concerning sex, his door was always open. At the same time he decried the lack of research concerning sex, all of which was the catalyst for the future that would turn his tawdry lifestyle and attempts at sex with anyone at any cost, into his worldwide reputation as a scientific genius. Just like the German Magnus Hirschfeld who was known for his years of sexual research in Germany, an occasion for Hirschfeld to fulfill his own sexual desires [one of his acolytes was the writer Christopher Isherwood] (15), and Baden-Powell, the inventor of the Boy Scouts so close to the heart of Kinsey, yet a man reported to have had sex with an incalculable number of boys, in South Africa and India, so too was Kinsey on the road to limitless orgasms, with "subjects" chosen from a population of hundreds. The difference was that Kinsey also had a scientific side to him, one that has supposedly made his work faultless in precision. We must perhaps judge a man by his contributions to the advancement of his fellow men, and not his private life.

Sir Laurence Olivier, whose private life would make some cringe (8), and who had used his fame and position to entice lads onto his casting coach, nonetheless produced and starred in *Hamlet*--so do we really need to know that went on backstage? Such is our conundrum with Alfred Kinsey, a man who ordered his wife home while he partied with all the enthusiasm of a Messalina.

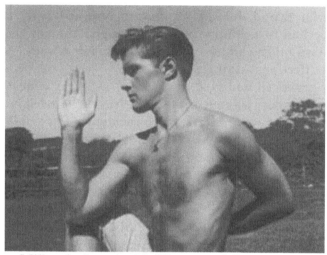

William Miller, intimate with Kinsey and Somerset Maugham.

Several hang-ups have always been part and parcel of an American's life, perhaps the inner belief in Calvinist hard work that could be jinxed by too much sexual felicity. During my years in Rome I was amazed at the ease with which Italians accepted their sexuality. I saw boys parade around their homes and have breakfast in their briefs, *served* by doting mothers and sisters, while at the beach young lads would pull down their swim suits to compare fully-erect phalluses and pubic bush growth, the adults around them sleeping like sated seals. My own childhood was partially destroyed by Mormon obscurantism, although my buddy at the time, an Eastern Yale boy, was not more enlightened than I: he had promised God he would never masturbate again if Yale accepted him; it did, and he held out for three whole days. In reality, American sexual beliefs were still dominated by Victorian ideals, and that into the 1920s and '30s (8).

Kinsey had had a lifetime of unanswered questions, and the more he interviewed his students, the more he discovered the scope of their, and his, ignorance. Doctors who should have led the way to enlightenment hammered nail after nail in the coffin of sex, providing lists of the mortal diseases whose roots sprang from self-abuse, doctors who labeled homosexuals as hermaphrodites, perversions that Nature had embodied with both sexes.

The more Kinsey delved into the subject of sex, in small groups that soon developed into full conferences, the more he decided to do something about his and his students' ignorance on the subject. He was one of the first to take an interest in endocrinology, and became convinced that there was a male sex hormone that would be the answer to all outstanding questions. [In 1889 a Harvard professor injected himself with an elixir derived from dog testicles. He felt more vigorous, but abandoned his research due to the criticism of fellow professors. Two scientists received the Nobel Prize of 1939 for isolating testosterone, and its vital role in sex became clearer in the 1950s and '60s, years after Kinsey had predicted the existence of the hormone.]

In 1937 Kinsey gave a lecture in which he introduced a slide showing a real vagina being penetrated by a real phallus, and told the students exactly what was going on pleasure-wise [going so far as to tell the boys to use spit as a lubricant--boys who probably hadn't as yet discovered that saliva was great in simply jerking off]. He certainly had the boys' dry-throated attention, their dicks just as certainly rock-hard, as this was the first vagina and the first fully-deployed phallus they had ever seen, outside of their own.

By 1938 Kinsey was no longer handsome, but thanks to his classes and conferences he no longer had to go looking for people for sex. People now pursued him, an earth-shattering difference in the life of a man set on having a maximum number of orgasms [the porn star Al Parker had had the same ambition (4)]. The more he freed his students from their sexual ignorance, the more they opened up their minds and bodies to him, all of which makes me wonder if Hugh Hefner ever had it so good?

In 1939 he went on the first of many trips to Chicago to visit the gay community that was anonymously established in big cities to escape attention. He appears to have taken great care of the gays and was probably sincere in the friendships he formed, as his letters to the boys there demonstrated true fondness for them. He invited several to his home in Indiana to meet his family, all of whom he treated with great respect. His weak spot, one present in many homosexuals, was his difficulty in accepting effeminate boys whose effeminacy, he told them, was learned, and so advised them to un-learn it. It's true that many homosexuals desperately want to be men in the image of heterosexual men, and so have little tolerance for those who lack outward virility. Fortunately many homosexuals, like Tim Cook, like myself, are so convinced of the great chance we have in being able to love other men--loving of their masculine beauty, masculine intelligence and tenderness--that we can overcome the loathing of homophobic heterosexuals, not as lucky as we.

Sexually, Kinsey took advantage of his outings in Chicago, certainly blowing and being blown, certainly sauna sex, perhaps glory-hole interludes and anal intercourse [all of which are integral part of his research notes], and like all the homosexuals he frequented he could spend the night slumming and the next day act as if, when he came across the men of the evening before, he hadn't received their semen in some intimate part of his body.

Back on campus student interest in his classes and research had grown to the point that two fraternities told him that 100% of their members would enter into his program. Thanks to his knowledge and fatherly ways with boys, he would woo, what?, some?/many?/most? into his bed, drawn by their beauty while they, as with Alcibiades and his liaison with the homely Socrates, were drawn to his experience and erudition (19).

In my book *Secret Societies* I go into the history of the Bloomsbury Set, where sex of unbelievable dimension was going on, in which some girls would mate with boys simply because the boys were the lovers of the men the girls really loved, and sleeping with the boys was a way of getting nearer to their true loves. It has been suggested that Kinsey's wife slept with the boys Kinsey slept with, as a way too of getting closer to her husband. At any rate, he passed her around to whoever took her fancy. He didn't care, and probably never had cared.

As his university courses were found not exactly ''proper'' by an increasingly larger number of faculty members, deeply jealous of the crowds that filled his classes and conferences, he took his research off campus. There are a huge number of foundations in America, and several came to his aid, the king of the mountain being the Rockefeller Foundation. Kinsey had to meet many of its people to get his research funded, but as he had already collected a whopping 8,500 sexual histories [his proclaimed goal being 100,000], the needed money was forthcoming.

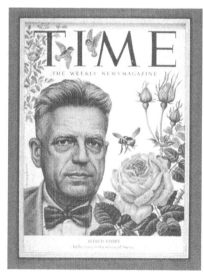

Time 1953

He hired interviewers, all sexually experienced, and when told by several that they were occasionally "attacked" by the interviewees, Kinsey told them to be passive, showing neither interest nor disdain, and he turned out to be right--there was apparently nothing that cooled ardor more than passivity. The men he hired were not exempt from his trying to have sex with them. One fled, confessing years later what Kinsey had blatantly tried to do to him--disgusting in the sense that the men had the choice of surrendering or losing their jobs.

Kinsey encouraged sex among the researchers themselves and regularly attended sexual encounters between his interviewees, and often watched people in action, his face inches from what was going on. Sexually he was insatiable. Photos were taken and films were made, and Kinsey assured one and all, on film, that all sexual problems could be surpassed with patience, desire and vaseline.

"Kinsey considered religion the source of most human misery," writes James Jones. "He had not the slightest doubt that religion was the root cause of sexual repression.'

Early on in his research Kinsey discovered that boys who did not finish school had the most orgasms, while college boys had the fewest. Working-class boys had orgasms through intercourse, college boys had most through masturbation.

When his research came to an end he had no problem finding an editor as they had been following his work for years and wanted a chance to capitalize on it. In fact, the competition became cutthroat, with everyone trying to lean on those they knew inside the Rockefeller Foundation, to get the sought-after grail. The book hit the stands in 1948, and all hell broke out.

200,000 hardback copies sold in just two months, at $6.50 [$65 today!] for 804 pages. Nothing leaked out concerning his homosexuality and, indeed, he was congratulated on the "ideal" 30-year-long marriage he had with his wife. Margaret Mead criticized him for his serious, puritanical stand, for nowhere did he state that sex was "fun". If the gal only knew! Amidst the euphoria of his success the Rockefeller Foundation accorded him $40,000 to continue his good works.

I read the book years later, far too late to help me confront my adolescent hang-ups, but the case studies fueled a huge number of orgasms, as did the drawings of naked cave men, at the time, in *National Geographic* magazines, nothing visible, of course, but it was all the world could offer in pornography then, and for me it was plenty.

A book of that nature caused huge discord in scientific circles, which apparently weighed heavily on Kinsey as everyone who knew him found him exhausted and all said he'd aged well beyond his years. James Jones compared him to the mainspring of a watch that was wound tighter and tighter. At the same time, flush with money, he enlarged his research team for the express purpose of increasing the number of his sexual partners. Sex between them all became an unsaid obligation if they wished to remain. It was like Andy Warhol's Factory (4) where everyone was forced to participate in the orgies. One researcher did stress that Kinsey was *also* having sex with women.

In 1948 Kinsey decided he would like to see exactly how men climaxed in masturbation. He hired a 17-year-old hustler, an extremely beautiful boy, to organize a session that would involve 2,000 men. The line of participants, each receiving $2, wound down the street and around the block, and although they didn't get the 2,000, they did film hundreds of orgasms [sheets were placed on the floor of the room where the "research" took place, and replaced when soaked through]. The "beautiful boy" had come through with lots of very young beauties, for which he was paid $2 a head. [At around the same time Pier Paolo Pasolini was recorded as having lined up 25 boys on a beach outside Rome--the beach where he was later murdered--and jerked off each one, considered the ultimate in eroticism by those who hadn't heard of Kinsey's doings.]

By the way, the session did prove that most men's sperm did not shoot out as seen in porn films, but rather "dribbled" over their fists.

Kinsey had many contacts with homosexuals who were stressed out of their minds by their "dirty" conduct. He assured them that they had nothing to feel guilty about, and to those trying to become "normal", he told them that it was as easy for a heterosexual to become homosexual as a homosexual to become heterosexual. Meaning: Don't even try.

As said at the beginning of this chapter, Kinsey was noted for being stubborn, and thanks to the incredible success of his book his stubbornness was reinforced, and his way of handling Foundation members who sought information concerning the reliability of his statistics [statistics put in question by scientists everywhere] was not always gentle, although he did usually try, at first, an amiable approach, often inviting Foundation members to his home for dinner. How much Foundation trustees knew about what went on in Kinsey's research center between the researchers, or how he employed underage lads to procure other underage lads for mass sessions in masturbation, is not known. What is known is that these men, for the most part, were Christian family fathers, who would certainly have put the brakes on if they'd had an inkling of the no-holds-barred acts Kinsey was filming. Opposition came from groups that disputed Kinsey's statistics, scientists who thought he had bent the outcome of his interviews to support the results Kinsey himself wished to obtain. In truth, Kinsey had to battle hard against a huge array of opponents, but he did so brilliantly, proof being that the Foundation continued to fund him, even if the stress greatly harmed him physically.

He was convinced that he was brilliant, and that his research was valid, but no matter how extraordinary he found himself, I wonder if he could have imagined that, 60 years after the publication of *Sexual Behavior in the Human Male* his name would still be familiar to every educated household in the world?

Yet he lived in an inner hell, one described in excruciating detail by James Jones, when Kinsey, unable to inflict enough pain on himself through introducing objects into his urethra, tied one end of a rope around his testicles, the other around an overhead pipe, climbed on a chair, and then jumped off.

His book, and the book that followed on female sexuality, caused so much unrest and dispute that funding dried up, and he spent what remained of his time on earth chasing nickels and dimes to keep his research center open, and for the first time he charged fees for his conferences.

He traveled to Rome where only the sexual underground interested him, and the only monument that caught his attention was the Coliseum, at night, where sex took place, one of many sites favored by Gore Vidal [who knew and contributed to Kinsey's research] (9). He went to Portugal where he complained about not getting laid as often as he wished. Back home he went on with his research, until felled by a heart attack in 1956.

It could have been such a marvelous life. Like all the men who are great in my eyes, he used life and allowed life to use him, the very meaning of our existence. He had his research and the backing of his researchers, all faithful and accepting of his ways. Yet his inner demons pushed him to desecrate himself and his body, as T.E. Lawrence had done, Lawrence who should have died by a bullet in Damascus, before allowing himself to be whipped mercilessly by boys Lawrence paid to inflict the pain, and Kinsey should have died directly after the publication of the work that makes him famous to this day, before stringing himself up by his balls.

ACKNOWLEDGEMENTS

A great many sources have been used in writing this book, as well as hundreds of pages downloaded from the Net, and *Wikipedia* was consulted hundreds of times in order to gather and verify facts. One book was especially useful, *God's Doodle, The Life and Times of the Penis*, by Tom Hickman, 2012, a superb work filled with information, as well as James H.

Jones's excellent *Alfred C. Kinsey, a life*, 1997, upon which I based my chapter on Kinsey.

FINAL CURTAIN

I'm not going into the ravages of age so as not to disorient young readers, whom I simply advise to live their sexuality to the hilt.

Caesar revealed what for him would be the perfect end to Brutus, an excerpt taken from my book *Roman Homosexuality*: ''The Ides of March, the 15th, came and we have the Shakespearean warning as he made his way to the senate, 'Beware of the Ides of March Caesar!' 'The Ides of March have come,' was Caesar's answer. 'Yes,' said the soothsayer, 'but have not gone!' The night before, Caesar had dined with his purported son, Brutus, and the topic of the best possible demise was raised. Caesar had replied, 'For me, a sudden, unexpected death!' ''

Such a rapid and unexpected death could come, if one is supremely lucky, in what the French call *la mort d'amour*, what we call death in the saddle, or when giving oneself pleasure, which happens far more often than one imagines, and always brings the grudging acknowledgement by those who find the lucky stiff that going that way, in truth, is the only way to go.

POSTSCRIPT

Phallic worship begins at birth, when the child in ancient times was laid at the father's feet and the tiny blanket opened. At the sight of the scepter the father would gratefully raise the boy above his head, to full approval of those attending, for the scepter was the incontestable emblem that the child would grow into an oak, tall, strong and virile, who would be the power over the household were he born in a village, over a domain were his parents noble, or over the world itself, as was the destiny of Cyrus, Alexander and Caesar. He had the potential of becoming the intellectual Nietzsche had been, an artist like da Vinci and Michelangelo, an historian as was Herodotus, a writer like Homer and Shakespeare, a mathematician, an explorer, the first man to step foot on Mars. The father would now live eternally--a man's single and *only* true promise of an afterlife--through the thighs of the son in his arms, a boy who will perpetuate his name and his place in the universe, until the universe no longer exists. It is this, the covenant of the boy and his scepter, in times barbarous and in times enlightened. It is this the immutable promise of the phallus.

SOURCES

(1) See my book *Michael Hone, His World, His Loves*.

(2) See my book *Exploration Giants*.

(3) See my book *The Garden of Allah*.

(4) See my book *HUSTLERS*.

(5) See my book *Henry III*.

(6) See my book *Renaissance Homosexuality*.

(7) See my book *Hadrian and Antinous*.

(8) See my book *Christ Has His John, I Have My George*.

(9) See my book *American Homosexual Giants*.

(10) See my book *Louis XIII*.

(11) See my book *Cesare Borgia*.

(12) See my book *TROY*.

(13) See my book *Cellini*.

(14) See my book *SPARTA*.

(15) See my book *Prussian Homosexuality*.

(16) See my book *Greek Homosexuality*.

(17) See my book *Venice*.

(18) See my book *Sacred Band*.

(19) See my book *Alcibiades*.

The major sources for the Greek and Roman segment of this book are the following:

<u>Aelianus</u> was a Roman author and teacher of rhetoric who spoke and wrote in Greek.

<u>Aeschylus</u>, of whom 7 out of perhaps 90 plays have survived. His gravestone celebrated his heroism during the victory against the Persians at Marathon and *not his plays*, proof of the extraordinary importance of Greek survival against the barbarians (sadly, he lost his brother at Marathon). He is said to have been a deeply religious person, dedicated to Zeus. As a boy he worked in a vineyard until Dionysus visited him in a dream and directed him to write plays. One of his plays supposedly divulged too much about the Eleusinian Mysteries and he was nearly stoned to death by the audience. He had to stand trial but pleaded ignorance. He got off when the judges learned of the death of his brother at Marathon and when Aeschylus showed the wounds he and a second brother had received at Marathon too, the second brother left with but a stump in place of his hand. In one of his later plays, Pericles was part of the chorus. The subjects of his plays often concerned Troy and the Persian Wars, Marathon, Salamis and Xerxes (Xerxes is accused of losing the war due to hubris; his building of the bridge over the Hellespont was a show of arrogance the gods found unacceptable). In *Seven against Thebes* he too tells about Oedipus' two sons. This time the boys agree to become kings of Thebes on alternate years. Naturally, when the time comes for them to change places the king in place

refuses, which leads to both boys killing each other. *Agamemnon* is an excellent retelling of the Trojan War, as Agamemnon sails home to be murdered by his wife Clytemnestra. In *The Libation Bearers* Agamemnon's boy Orestes returns home to destroy his father's assassins, Clytemnestra and her lover Aegisthus. In *The Eumenides* (the Kindly Spirits) Orestes is chased by the Furies for having killed his mother. He takes shelter with Apollo who decides, with Athena, to try the boy before a court. The vote is a tie, but Athena, preaching the importance of reason and understanding, acquits him. She then changes the terrible Furies into sweet Eumenides.

Anacreon was born in 582 B.C. and was known for his drinking songs.

Andocides was implicated in the Hermes scandal and saved his skin by turning against Alcibiades in a speech that has come down to us called, what else?, *Against Alcibiades*.

Appian, who lived during the reigns of Trajan and Hadrian, was a Roman historian of Greek origin. He was a friend of Fronto, Marcus Aurelius' tutor and, perhaps, lover. He left his book, *Roman History*, which describes, among other events, the Roman civil wars.

Aristophanes, my preferred playwright, is, naturally, the father of comedy. He wrote perhaps 40 plays of which 11 remain. He was feared by all: Plato states that it was his play *The Clouds* the root of the trial that cost Socrates his life. Nearly nothing is known about him other than what he himself revealed in his works. Playwrights were obliged to be conservative because part of each play was funded by a wealthy citizen, an honor for the citizen and a caveat for the author. He was an exponent of make-love-not-war who saw his country go from its wonderful defeat of the Persians to its end at the hands of the Spartans. Along with Alcibiades and Socrates, Aristophanes is featured in Plato's *The Symposium* in which he is gently mocked, proof that he was considered, even by those he poked fun at, as affable. *The Acharnians* highlights the troubles the Athenians went through after the death of Pericles and their defeat at the hands of Sparta. *The Peace* focuses on the Peace of Nicias. *Lysistrata* tells about the plight of women trying to bring about peace in order to prevent the sacrifice of their sons during war, occasioning the world's first sex strike. When Athens lost its freedom to Sparta, Aristophanes stopped writing plays.

Athenaeus lived in the times of Marcus Aurelius. His *Deipnosopistae* is a banquet conversation *à la Platon* during which conversations on every possible subject took place, filling fifteen books that have come down to us.

Ausonius was a Latin poet and teacher of rhetoric, around 350 B.C.

Bion was a Greek philosopher known for his diatribes, satires and attacks on religion. He lived around 300 B.C.

Cassius Dio, 155 A.D. to 235 A.D., was a noted historian who wrote in Greek and published a history of Rome in 80 volumes, many of which have survived, giving modern historians a detailed look into his times.

Cicero was born in 106 B.C. and murdered by Mark Antony in 43 B.C. Michael Grant said it all when he wrote, ''the influence of Cicero upon the history of European literature and ideas greatly exceeds that of any other prose writer in any language.''

Cornelius Nepos was a Roman friend of Cicero. Most of what he wrote was lost, so what we know comes through passages of his works in the books of other historians.

Ctesias was a Greek historian from Anatolian Caria, and the physican of Artaxerxes, whom he accompanied in his war against his brother Cyrus the Younger. He wrote a book on India, *Indica* and Persia, *Persica*. The fragments we have of his writing come to us through Diodorus Siculus and Plutarch.

Diodorus Siculus lived around 50 B.C. and wrote *Historical Library*, consisting of forty volumes.

Diogenes of Sinope (aka Diogenes the Cynic) comes to use through extracts of his writing passed on by others, as nothing he wrote has survived. He had a truly remarkable life, at first imprisoned for debasing the coins his father, a banker, minted. Afterwards he pled poverty, sleeping in a huge ceramic jar, walking the streets of Athens during the day with a lighted lamp, saying he was in search of an honest man, and teasing Plato by noisily eating through his lectures (later Plato claimed he was ''a Socrates gone mad''.) On a voyage he was captured and sold as a slave in Crete to a Corinthian who was so entranced by his intelligence that he made him his sons' teacher. It was in his master's household that he grew old and died. Plutarch tells us he met Alexander the Great while Diogenes was staring at a pile of bones. In answer to Alexander's question he said he was searching for the bones of Alexander's father, but could not distinguish them from those of a slave. To which Alexander supposedly said that if he couldn't be Alexander he would choose to be Diogenes. He was the first man ever to claim to be ''a citizen of the world.'' He urinated on people, defecated where he would and masturbated in public, about which he said, ''If only I could banish hunger by rubbing my belly.'' The word cynic meant dog-like, and when someone questioned him about it he said he too was dog-like because he licked those who helped him, barked at those who didn't, and bit his enemies. Rogers and Hart wrote these lyrics about him: There was an old zany/who lived in a tub; he had so many flea-bites/he didn't know where to rub.

Eupolis lived around 430 B.C. An Athenian poet who wrote during the Peloponnesian Wars.

Euripides may have written 90 plays of which 18 survive. His approach was a study of the inner lives of his personages, the predecessor of Shakespeare. Due to his stance on certain subjects, he thought it best to leave Athens voluntarily rather than suffer an end similar to that of

Socrates. An example: ''I would prefer to stand three times to confront my enemies in battle rather than bear a single child!'' He was born on the island of Salamis, of Persian-War fame; in fact he was born on the very day of the battle. His youth was spent in athletics and dance. Due to bad marriages with unfaithful wives, he withdrew to Salamis where he wrote while contemplating sea and sky. When Sparta defeated Athens in war, it did not destroy the city-state: Plutarch states that this was thanks to one of Euripides' plays, *Electra*, put on for the Spartans in Athens, a play they found so wonderful that they proclaimed that it would be barbarous to destroy a city capable of engendering men of the quality of Euripides. (The real reason was to preserve the city that had twice saved Greece from Persian victory.) Euripides was known for his love of Agathon, a youth praised for his beauty as well as for his culture, and would later become a playwright. Aristophanes mocked Euripides for loving Agathon long after he had left his boyhood behind him. (Remember, not everyone followed boy-love to the letter. The idea of men loving boys until they grew whiskers did not always hold true. Boys grown ''old'' could shave their chins and butts; some men just preferred other men, hairy or not; most men impregnated boys but other men adored being penetrated.) Plato says that Agathon had polished manners, wealth, wisdom and dispensed hospitality with ease and refinement.

Herodian wrote a history of Greece entitled *History of the Empire from the Death of Marcus*, in eight books. Thanks to him we learn a great deal about Elagabalus.

Herodotus was also contemporary to the events that interest us here. Cicero called him the Father of History, while Plutarch wrote that he was the Father of Lies. His masterpiece is *The Histories*, considered a chef-d'oeuvre, a work that the gods have preserved intact right up to our own day, a divine intervention that would not have surprised a believer like Herodotus (it's also a book I reread every year). Part of his work may have been derived from other sources (what historian's work isn't?) and the facts rearranged in an effort to give them dramatic force and please an audience. Much of what he did was based on oral histories, many of which themselves were based on early folk tales, highly suspect, naturally, in all their details. Aristophanes made fun of segments of his work and Thucydides called Herodotus a storyteller. Surprisingly little is known about his own life. For example, he writes lovingly about Samos, leading some to believe that he may have spent his youth there. Born near Ionia, he wrote in that dialect, learning it perhaps on Samos. He was his own best publicist, taking his works to festivals and games, such as the Olympic Games, and reading them to the spectators. As I've said, many people doubt that he actually went where he said he went and saw what he said he saw. But the same was true of Marco Polo who causes disbelief to this day simply because he never mentioned eating noodles in China or seeing the Great Wall or even drinking Chinese tea. But no historian, then as now, can write a book on ancient occurrences without referring to Herodotus' observations. An amusing example of recent discoveries that give credence to Herodotus is this: Herodotus wrote about a kind of giant ant, the size of a fox, living in India, in the desert, that dug up gold. This was ridiculed until the French ethnologist Peissel came upon a marmot living in today's Pakistan that burrows in the sand and has for generations brought wealth to the region by bringing up gold from its burrows. Peissel suggests that the original confusion came from the fact that the Persian word for marmot was similar to the word for mountain ant.

Isocrate was a student of Socrates who wrote a speech in the defense of Alcibiades during a trial that took place after his death.

Josephus, 37 A.D. to around 100 A.D., was a historian born in Jerusalem. He fought against the Romans and was captured by Vespasian who kept him as his interpreter and, later, Josephus even assumed the emperor's family name, becoming a citizen (Titus Flavius Josephus). A Jew, he turned against his people and helped Vespasian's son Titus to loot the Second Temple. His works include *The Jewish War* and *Antiquities of the Jews.*

Juvenal was a satirical poet who wrote *Satires*.

Lucan (Marcus Annaeus Lucanus) lived from 39 A.D. to 65 A.D., a short life due to his being ordered by Nero to commit suicide because of his role in the treasonous Piso conspiracy. In hopes of a pardon, he implicated his mother among others, all of whom followed him in death. He was a poet, a close friend of Nero until the emperor grew tired of him and his poetry, after which Lucan's writing became insulting, insults Nero was said to have ignored.

Lysias was extremely wealthy and contemporary with Alcibiades. He founded a new profession, logographer, which consisted of writing speeches delivered in law courts. One of his speeches was *Against Andocides*, another was *Against Alcibiades.*

Memmius was an orator and poet, and friend of Pompey but eventually went over to Caesar.

Mimnermus was born in Ionian Smyrna around 630 B.C. He wrote short love poems suitable for performance at drinking parties.

Myron of Priene is the author of a historical account of the First Messenian War.

Pausanias, a Greek historian and geographer, famous for his *Description of Greece*. He was contemporary with Hadrian and Marcus Aurelius. He's noted as being someone interested in everything, careful in his writing and scrupulously honest.

Phanocles lived during the time of Alexander the Great. He was the author of a poem on boy-love that described the love of Orpheus for Calais, and his death at the hands of Thracian women.

Philemon lived to be a hundred but alas only fragments of his works remain. He must have been very popular as he won numerous victories as a poet and playwright.

Pindar's great love was Theoxenus of Tenodos about whom he wrote: ''Whosoever, once he has seen the rays flashing from the eyes of Theoxenus, and is not shattered by the waves of desire, has a black heart forged of a cold flame. Like wax of the sacred bees, I melt when I look at the young limbs of boys.'' He lived around 500 B.C. and celebrated the Greek victories against the Persians at Salamis and Plataea. His home in Thebes became a must for his devotees.

Plato was a major source for this book, along with Xenophon, Thucydides and Plutarch. Plato's most famous work is the Allegory of the Cave. Humans in the cave have no other reality than the shadows they see on the walls. If they looked around they could see what was casting the shadows and by doing so gain additional knowledge. If they left the cave they would discover the sun, analogous to truth. If those who saw the sun reentered the cave and told the others, they would not be believed. There are thusly different levels of reality that only the wisest are able to see; the others remain ignorant. It's basically thanks to Plato and Xenophon that we know what we do about Socrates. Plato's perfect republic is ruled by the best (an aristocracy), headed by a philosopher king who guides his people thanks to his wisdom and reason. An inferior form of government, one that comes after an aristocracy, is a timocracy, ruled by the honorable. A timocracy is in the hands of a warrior class. Plato has Sparta in mind, but it's unclear how he could have found this form of government better than, for example, a democracy. The problem may be that we know, in reality, so little about Sparta. Next comes an oligarchy based on wealth, followed by a democracy, rule by just anyone and everyone. This degenerates into a tyranny, meaning a government of oppression, because of the conflict between the rich and the poor in a democracy.

Pliny the Younger was the Elder's nephew. He too witnessed the explosion of Vesuvius. He was a lawyer and a letter writer, many of which remain, vital historical sources of the times. His letters concerning Trajan are of special importance. Under Trajan he worked side by side with Suetonius.

Plutarch was born near Delphi around 46 A.D. to a wealthy family. He was married, and a letter to his wife even exists to this day. He had sons, the exact number unknown. He studied mathematics and philosophy in Athens and was known to have visited most of the major Greek sites mentioned in this book, as well as Rome. He personally knew the Emperors Trajan and

Hadrian, and became a Roman citizen. He was a high priest at Delphi and his duty consisted of interpreting the auguries of the Pythoness (no mean task). He wrote the *Lives of the Emperors* but alas only two of the lesser emperors survive. Another verily monumental work was *Parallel Lives of Greeks and Romans* of which twenty-three exist. His interest was the destinies of his subjects, how they made their way through the meanders of life. I too have a passionate interest in how men strive their wholes lives for success, only to be crushed, like Alcibiades, like Pericles, at the end. In explanation of his oeuvre Plutarch wrote that what interested him was not history but lives, and the Jekyll/Hyde struggle of virtue versus vice. A small jest, he went on, often reveals more than battles during which thousands die. His writings on Sparta, alongside those of Xenophon, are nearly all we possess concerning that extraordinary city-state. His major biographies are the *Life of Alexander* and the *Life of Julius Caesar.* Amusingly, Plutarch wrote a scathing review of Herodotus' work in which he stated that the great historian was fanatically biased in favor of the Greeks who could do, according to Herodotus, no wrong.

No gratitude can ever be enough for what this man has given us, although in the case of the Greeks we must never forget that he was writing *500 years after the events.*

Polybius, around 200 B.C. to 118 B.C. was a Greek historian whose *The Histories* covered the period from 264 to 146 B.C. He was a friend of Scipio Africanus. He details the ascent to empire of Rome, and was present at the destruction of Carthage.

Polyenus was a Macedonian known as a rhetorician and for his books on war strategies.

Sallust was a Roman historian and politician, 86 B.C. to about 35 B.C. One of his works concerned Catiline and he wrote *Histories* of which only fragments remain.

Seneca (Lucius Annaeus Seneca) lived around 4 B.C. to 65 A.D. He was the advisor of Caligula, Claudius and Nero who forced him to commit suicide for supposedly planning his overthrow. He is known for his philosophical essays, letters and tragedies.

Simonides of Ceos was a Greek poet born about 550 B.C. Besides his poems, he added four letters to the Greek alphabet.

Suetonius (Gaius Suetonius Tranquillus) lived around 69 A.D. to 123 A.D. He was a truly great Roman historian known for his *Twelve Caesars,* his only extant work. Pliny the Younger says that he was studious and totally dedicated to writing. He was highly favored by both Trajan, under whom he served as his secretary, and Hadrian who fired him for having an affair with the Empress Vibia Sabina.

Sophocles was the author of 123 plays of which 7 remain, notably *Oedipus* and *Antigone.* An Athenian born to a rich family just before the

Battle of Marathon, he was a firm supporter of Pericles. He fought alongside Pericles against Samos when the island attempted to become autonomous from Athens. He was elected as a magistrate during the Sicilian Expedition led by Alcibiades, and given for function the goal of finding out why the expedition had ended disastrously. Sophocles was always ready and willing to succumb to the charms of boys. Plutarch tells us that even at age 65 ''he led a handsome boy outside the city walls to have his way with him. He spread the boy's poor himation--a rectangular piece of cloth thrown over the left shoulder that drapes the body--upon the ground. To cover them both he spread his rich cloak. After Sophocles took his pleasure the boy took the cloak and left the himation for Sophocles. This misadventure was eventually known to all.'' He died at 90, some say while reciting a very long tirade from *Antigone* because he hadn't paused to take a breath. Another version has him choking on grapes, and a final one has him dying of happiness after winning the equivalent of our Oscar at a festival. The first of his trilogy--called the Theban plays--is *Oedipus the King*. Here the baby Oedipus--in a plot that goes back to Priam and Paris at the founding of Troy--is handed over to a servant to be killed in order to prevent the accomplishment of an oracle, an oracle stating that he will kill his father and marry his mother. He does both after solving the riddle of the sphinx (which creature becomes four-footed, then two-footed and finally three-footed?). His mother, when she finds out she's been bedding her own son, commits suicide and Oedipus blinds himself. In *Oedipus at Colonus* Oedipus dies and we learn more about his children Antigone, Polyneices and Eteocles. In *Antigone* Polyneices is accused of treason and killed. His body is thrown outside the city walls and the king forbids its burial, under pain of death. Antigone does so anyway and, faced with death, she commits suicide, followed by the king's son who was going to wed her, followed by the king's wife who couldn't face losing her precious son. (Whew!)

Tacitus, around 56 A.D. to 117 A.D., was a historian who wrote *Annals* and *Histories*, concerning Tiberius, Claudius, Nero and the Year of the Four Emperors. He is known for his insights into the psychology of his subjects.

Theocritus was a Sicilian and lived around 270 B.C. In his 7th Idyll Aratus is passionately in love with a lad. His 12th Idyll refers to Diocles who died saving the life of Philolaus, the boy he loved, and in whose honor kissing contests were held every spring at his tomb. In his 23rd Idyll a lover commits suicide because of unrequited love, warning his belovèd that one day he too will burn and weep for a cruel boy. Before hanging himself the lover kissed the doorpost from which he would attach the noose. The boy treated the corpse with disdain and went off to the gymnasium for a swim where a statue of Eros fell on him, coloring the water with his blood. In his

29th Idyll a lover warns his belovèd that he too will age and his beauty will lose its freshness. He is therefore advised to show more kindness as ''you will one day be desperate for a beautiful young man's attentions.'' Although lads are often disappointing, it is impossible not to fall madly in love with them. In the 30th Idyll the poet states that when a man grows old he should keep a distance from boys, but in his heart he knows that the only alternative to loving a boy is simply to cease to exist.

Theognis was born around 550 B.C. His poems consist of maxims and advice as to how to live life. Fortunately, a great deal of his work has come down to us, most of which is dedicated to his belovèd, the handsome Cyrnus.

Thucydides was an Athenian general and historian, contemporary with the events he described. What he wrote was based on what actually happened; there was no extrapolating; no divine intervention on the part of the gods as was the case with Plutarch. An example of this was his observation that birds and animals that ate plague victims died as a result, leading him to conclude that the disease had a natural rather than supernatural cause. His description of the plague has never been equaled, the plague that he himself caught while participating in the Peloponnesian War. He is thought to have died in 411 B.C., the date at which his writing suddenly stops. He admired Pericles and democracy but not the radical form found in Athens.

Tibullus died in 19 B.C. at the age of 36 but I've not learned how. He was a Latin poet who lost most of his estate to the confiscations of Marc Antony and Augustus. Why, I know not.

Tyrtaeus, a rare Spartan writer, left us an account of the Second Messenian War. The purpose of his poetry was to inspire Spartan support of the Spartan state. Athenians claimed he was of Athenian birth. Pausanias maintained that the Athenians had sent him to Sparta as an insult, because he was both crazy, lame and had one eye. Herodotus wrote that he was only one of two foreigners to be given Spartan citizenship.

Xenophon, born near Athens in 430 B.C., was a historian and general. His masterpieces are *The Peloponnesian Wars* and *Anabasis*. He loved Sparta and served under Spartan generals during the Persian Wars. Like the Spartans, he believed in oligarchic rule, rule by the few, be they the most intelligent or wealthy or militarily acute. He spent a great deal of time in Persia alongside Cyrus the Younger who raised an army, among whom were Xenophon's 10,000 and other mercenaries (all of which is the subject of *Anabasis*). After Cyrus' death Xenophon and his ten thousand made their way back home, the breathtaking account of which ends his *Anabasis*. The Athenians exiled him when he fought with the Spartans against Athens but the Spartans offered him an estate where he wrote his works. His banishment may have been revoked thanks to his son Gryllus who brilliantly fought and died for Athens.

Other Sources:

Abbott Jacob, *History of Pyrrhus*, 2009
Ady, Cecilia, *A History of Milan under the Sforza*, 1907.
Aggleton, Peter, *Men Who Sell Sex*, 1999.
Aldrich and Wotherspoon, *Who's Who in Gay and Lesbian History*, 2001.
Aldrich, Robert, *The Seduction of the Mediterranean*, 1993.
Andress, David, *The Terror*, 2005.
Aristophanes, Bantam Drama, 1962.
Aronson, Marc, *Sir Walter Ralegh*, 2000.
Baglione, *Caravaggio*, circa 1600.
Baker Simon, *Ancient Rome*, 2006.
Barber, Richard, *The Devil's Crown--Henry II and Sons*, 1978.
Barber, Stanley, *Alexandros*, 2010.
Bawlf, Samuel, *The Secret Voyage of Sir Francis Drake*, 2003.
Beachy, Robert, *Gay Berlin*, 2014. Marvelous.
Bellori, *Caravaggio*, circa 1600.
Bentley, Jim, *Last Time I drew A Crowd*, 2005.
Bergreen Laurence, *Over the Edge of the World – Magellan*.
Bierman, John, *Dark Safari, Henry Morton Stanley*, 1990.
Bonnard, Marc and Michel Schouman, *Histoire du Pénis*, 1999.
Boswell, John, *Christianity, Social Tolerance, and Homosexuality*, 1980.
Boswell, John, *Same-Sex Unions*, 1994.
Bowers, Scotty, *Full Service*, 2012.
Boyd, Douglas, *April Queen*, 2004.
Boyles, David, *Blondel's Song*, 2005.
Bradford, Ernle, *Thermopylae*, 1980.
Bramly, Serge, *Leonardo*, 1988. A wonderful book.
Brenot, Philipe, *In Praise of Masturbation*, 1997.
Bret, David, *Clark Gable*, 2007.
Bret, David, *Errol Flynn, Gentleman Hellraiser*, 2004,
Bret, David, *Joey Stefano*, 2015.
Bret, David, *Valentino*, 1998.
Bret, Davis, *Trailblazers*, 2009.
Bull, Lew, *Memoirs of a Hustler*, 2010.
Burg, B.R., *Gay Warriors*, 2002.
Bury and Meiggs, *A History of Greece*, 1975.
Calimach, Andrew, *Lover's Legends*, 2002.
Callow, Simon, *Charles Laughton*, 1995.
Capote, A Reader, Abacus, 1989.

Carpenter, Edward, *The Intermediate Sex*, 1912.

Carroll, Stuart, *Martyrs & Murderers, The Guise Family*, 2009.

Carry Peter, *True History of the Kelly Gang*, 2000.

Carson, H.A., *a thousand and one night stands*, 2001.

Carter, David, *Stonewall*, 2004.

Cartledge, Paul, *Alexander the Great*, 2004.

Cate, Curtis, *Friedrich Nietzsche*, 2003.

Cavel Benjamin, *Rumble, Young Man, Rumble*, 2003.

Cellini, Benvenuto, *The Autobiography of Benvenuto Cellini*.

Ceram, C.W., *Gods, Graves and Scholars*, 1951.

Chamberlin, E.R. *The Fall of the House of Borgia*, 1974.

Clark, Adrian and Jeremy Dronfield, *Queer Saint, Peter Watson*, 2015.

Clark, Gerald, *Capote*, 1988.

Cliff, Nigel, *The Last Crusade, The Epic Voyages of Vasco da Gama*, 2011.

Cloulas Ivan, *The Borgia*, 1989.

Conner, Clifford, *Jean Paul Marat*, 2012.

Cooper, John, *The Queen's Agent*, 2011.

Cowan, Thomas, *Gay Men and Women Who Enriched the World*, 1988/

Crompton, Louis, *Byron and Greek Love*, 1985.

Crompton, Louis, *Homosexuality and Civilization*, 2003.

Crouch, David, *William Marshal*, 1990.

Crowley, Roger, *Empires of the Sea*, 2008. Marvelous.

Curtis Cate, *Friedrich Nietzsche*, 2002.

Dale, Richard, *Who Killed Sir Walter Ralegh?*, 2011.

Dalrymple, William, *The Last Mughal*, 2006.

Davidson, James, *Courtesans and Fishcakes*, 1998.

Daniéliu, Alain, *The Phallus*, 1993,

Davidson, James, *The Greeks and Greek Love*, 2007.

Davidson, Michael, *The World, The Flesh and Myself*, 1977.

Davis, John Paul, *The Gothic King, Henry III*, 2013.

Dorais, Michel, *Rent Boys*, 2002,

Dover K.J. *Greek Homosexuality*, 1978

Duby, George, *William Marshal*, 1985.

Edmonson, Roger, *Boy in the Sand, Casey Donovan*, 1998.

Edmonson, Roger, *CLONE, The Life and Legend of Al Parker*, 2000.

Eisler, Benita, *BYRON Child of Passion, Fool of Fame*, 2000. Wonderful.

Ellmann, Richard, *Oscar Wilde*, 1987.

Erlanger, Philippe, *Buckingham*, 1951.

Erlanger, Philippe, *The King's Minion*, 1901.

Escoffier, Jeffrey, *Bigger Than Life*, 2009.

Evans, Robert, *The Kid Stays in the Picture*, 1994.

Everitt Anthony, *Augustus*, 2006

Everitt Anthony, *Cicero*, 2001.

Everitt Anthony, *Hadrian*, 2009

Fagles, Robert, *The Iliad*, 1990.

Fiore, Carlo, *The Brando I Knew*, 1974.

Forellino, Antonio, *Michelangelo*, 2005. Beautiful reproductions.

Fothergill, Brian, *Beckford of Fonthill*, 1979.

Fraser, Antonia, *The Gunpowder Plot*, 1996.

Frieda, Leonie, *Catherine de Medici*, 2003. Wonderful.

Friedman, David, *A Mind of Its Own*, 2001.

Gaylord, Martin, *Michelangelo: His Epic Life*, 2015.

Gillingham, John, *Richard the Lionheart*, 1978.

Gilmore, John, *Laid Bare*, 1997.

Goldsworthy Adrian, *Caesar*, 2006

Goldsworthy Adrian, *The Fall of Carthage*, 2000

Goodman Rob and Soni Jimmy, *Rome's Last Citizen*, 2012.

Goodwin, Robert, *SPAIN*, 2015.

Gore-Browne, Robert, *Lord Bothwell*, 1937.

Gordon, Richard, *The Alarming History of Sex*, 1996.

Graham-Dixon Andrew, *Caravaggio, A Life Sacred and Profane*, 2010.

Grant Michael, *History of Rome*, 1978

Graves, Robert, *Greek Myths*, 1955.

Gray, George, *The Children's Crusade*, (no date).

Grazia Sebastian de, *Machiavelli in Hell*, 1989.

Grèce, Michel de, *Le Vol du Régent*, 2008.

Guicciardini, *Storie fiorentine (History of Florence)*, 1509.

Halperin David M. *One Hundred Years of Homosexuality*, 1990.

Harris Robert, *Imperium*, 2006.

Harris, Frank, *My Life and Loves*, 1925.

Herodotus, *The Histories*, Penguin Classics.

Hesiod and Theognis, Penguin Classics, 1973.

Hibbard, Allen, *Paul Bowles*, 1993.

Hibbert Christopher, *Florence, the Biography of a City*, 1993.

Hibbert Christopher, *The Borgias and Their Enemies*, 2009.

Hibbert, Christopher, *Florence, the Biography of a City*, 1993.

Hibbert, Christopher, *The Days of the French Revolution*, 1981.

Hibbert, Christopher, *The Great Mutiny India 1857*, 1978. Fabulous.

Hibbert, Christopher, *The Rise and Fall of the House of Medici*, 1974.

Hickman, Tom, *God's Doodle*, 2012.

Hicks, Michael, *Richard III*, 2000.

Hine, Daryl, *Puerilities*, 2001.

Hirst, Michael, *The Tudors*, 2007.

Hochschild, Adam, *King Leopold's Ghost*, 1999.

Hofler, Robert, *Party Animals*, 2010.

Hofler, Robert, *The Man Who Invented Rock Hudson*, 2005.

Hogan, Steve, *Completely Queer, Gay and Lesbian Encyclopedia*, 1998.
Holland Tom, *Rubicon*, 2003
Hughes Robert, *Rome*, 2011
Hughes-Hallett, *Heroes*, 2004.
Hughes, Robert, *Rome*, 2011.
Hughes, Robert, *The Fatal Shore*, 1987.
Hulot, Frédéric, *Suffren, l'Amiral Satan*, 1994.
Hutchinson, Robert, *Elizabeth's Spy Master*, 2006.
Hutchinson, Robert, *House of Treason*, 2009.
Hutchinson, Robert, *Thomas Cromwell*, 2007.
Isherwood, Charles, *The Life and Death of Joey Stefano*, 1996.
Isherwood, Christopher, *Christopher and His Kind*, 1976.
Isherwood, Christopher, *Diaries*, vol. one, 2011.
Jack Belinda, *Beatrice's Spell*, 2004.
James, Callum, *My Dear KJ...* edited by James, 2015.
Jeal, Tim, *Explorers of the Nile*, 2011. Wonderful.
Jeal, Tim, *STANLEY*, 2007. All of Jeal's books are must-reads.
Jeffers, H. Paul, Sal Mineo, *His Life, Murder and Mystery*, 2000.
Johnson, Marion, *The Borgias*, 1981.
Jones, James H., *Alfred C. Kinsey, a life*, 1997.
Kagan, Donald, *The Peloponnesian War*, 2003.
Kanfer, Stefan, *Marlon Brando*, 2008.
Katz, Jonathan Ned, *Love Stories*, 2001.
Kearns, Michael, *The Truth is Bad Enough*, 2012,
Kelly, Ian, *Casanova: Actor Lover Priest Spy*, 2008.
Knecht, Robert, *The French Religious Wars 1562-98*, 2002.
Köhler, Joachim, *Zarathustra's Secret*, 1989.
Korda, Michael, *HERO The Life and Legend of Lawrence of Arabia*, 2010.
Lacey, Robert, *Henry VIII*, 1972.
Lacy, Robert, *Sir Walter Ralegh*, 1973.
Lahr, John, *Prick Up Your Ears, The Biography of Joe Orton*, 1978
Lahr, John, *Tennessee Williams, Mad Pilgrimage of the Flesh*, 2014.
Lambert Gilles *Caravaggio*, 2007.
Landucci, Luca, *A Florentine Diary*, around 1500, a vital source.
LaRue, Chi Chi, *Making it Big*, 1997.
Lawday, David, *Danton*, 2009.
Lawday, David, *Napoleon's Master,* 2007.
Lev, Elizabeth, *The Tigress of Forli*, 2011. Wonderfully written.
Levy, Buddy, *Conquistador*, 2009
Levy, Buddy, *River of Darkness*, 2011. Fabulous.
Lévy, *Edmond, Sparte, 1979.*
Lewis, Bernard, *The Assassins*, 1967.
Livy, *Rome and the Mediterranean.*

Livy, *The War with Hannibal*

Loomis, Stanley, *Paris in the Terror*, 1986.

Lubkin Gregory, *A Renaissance Court*, 1994.

Lyons, Mathew, *The Favourite*, 2011.

Macintyre, Ben, *The Man Who Would Be King*, 2004.

Mackay, James, *In My End is My Beginning, Mary Queen of Scots*, 1999.

Mackay, John Henry, *The Hustler*, 2002.

Malye, Jean, *La Véritable Histoire d'Alcibiade*, 2009.

Manchester William, *A World Lit Only By Fire*, 1993

Mancini, *Caravaggio*, circa 1600.

Mann, William, *Men Who Love Men*, 2007.

Mann, William, *The Men from the Boys*, 1998.

Mann, William, *Wisecracker*, 1998.

Manso, Peter, *Brando*, 1994.

Marchand, Leslie, *Byron*, 1971.

Martines, Lauro, *April Blood-Florence and the Plot against the Medici*, 2003.

Matyszak Philip, *Mithridates the Great*, 2008

McBrien, William, *Cole Porter*, 2000.

McCann, Graham, *Rebel Males*, 1991.

McGilligan, Patrick, *A Double Life--George Cukor*, 1991.

McLynn, Frank, *Richard and John, Kings of War*, 2007. Fabulous.

McLynn, *Marcus Aurelius*, 2009.

McLynn, *STANLEY, The making of an African explorer*, 1989.

McNamara, Robert P., *The Times Square Hustler*, 1994.

Meier, Christian, *Caesar*, 1996.

Merritt, Rich, *Secrets of a Gay Marine Porn Star*, 2005.

Meyer G.J. *The Borgias, The Hidden History*, 2013.

Meyer, G.J. *The Tudors*, 2010.

Meyer, Jack, *Alcibiades*, 2009.

Miles Richard, *Ancient Worlds*, 2010.

Miles Richard, *Carthage Must be Destroyed*, 2010

Miller, David, *Richard the Lionheart*, 2003.

Minichiello, Victor and John Scott, *Male Sex Work and Society*, 2014.

Moore Lucy, *Amphibious Thing*, 2000.

Moote, Lloyd, *Louis XIII, The Just*, 1989.

Mortimer, Ian, *1415, Henry V's Year of Glory*, 2009.

Nicholl, Charles, *The Reckoning*, 2002.

Niven, David, *Bring on the Empty Horses*, 1975.

Niven, David, *The Moon's a Balloon*, 1971.

Noel Gerard, *The Renaissance Popes*, 2006.

Norton, Rictor, *My Dear Boy, Gay Love Letters*, 1998.

O'Hara, Scott, *Autopornography, A Memoir of Life in the Lust Lane*, 1997.

Oosterhuis, Harry, *Homosexuality and Male Bonding*, 1991.

Opper Thorsten, *Hadrian*, 2008
Ostrow, Steve, *Live at the Continental*, 2007.
Paladilhe, Dominique, *Le Prince de Condé*, 2005.
Paring, Justin, *The life and times of Samuel Steward*, 2010.
Parini, Jay, *Empire of Self, A Life of Gore Vidal*, 2015.
Parish, James Robert, *The Hollywood Book of Death*, 2002.
Parker, Derek, *Cellini*, 2003, the book is beautifully written.
Parker, Peter, *Isherwood A Life*, 2004,
Pascal, Jean Claude, *L'Amant du Roi*, 1991.
Payne, Robert and Nihita Romanoff, *Ivan the Terrible*, 2002.
Pearce, Joseph, *The Unmasking of Oscar Wilde*, 2000.
Pernot, Michel, *Henri III*, Le Roi Décrié, 2013, Excellent book.
Petitfils, Jean-Christian, *Louis XIII*, 2008, wonderful.
Peyrefitte, Roger, *Alexandre*, 1979.
Plimpton, George, *Truman Capote*, 1998.
Plutarch's Lives, Modern Library.
Pollard, J., *Warwick the Kingmaker*, 2007.
Polybius, *The Histories*
Porter, Darwin & Roy Moseley, *Damn You, Scarlett O'Hara*, 2011.
Porter, Darwin and Danforth Prince, *Pink Triangle*, 2014.
Porter, Darwin, *Brando Unzipped*, 2004.
Porter, Darwin, *Howard Hughes*, 2010.
Porter, Darwin, *Paul Newman*, 2009.
Read, Piers Paul, *The Templars*, 1999.
Reed, Jeremy, *The Dilly*, 2014.
Reid, B.L., *The Lives of Roger Casement*, 1976.
Renucci Pierre, *Caligula*, 2000.
Reston, James, *Warriors of God, Richard and the Crusades*, 2001.
Rice, Edward, *Captain Sir Richard Francis Burton*, 1990.
Ridley, Jasper, *The Tudor Age*, 1998.
Robb Peter, M – *The Man Who Became Caravaggio*, 1998.
Robb Peter, *Street Fight in Naples*, 2010.
Robb, Peter, *Street Fight in Naples*, 2010.
Rocco, Antonio, *Alcibiade Enfant à l'Ecole*, 1630.
Rocke Michael, *Forbidden Friendships*, 1996, both indispensible and
Roen, Paul, *High Camp*, 1994.
Rolfe, Frederick, Letters to Charles Kains Jackson, *My Dear KJ...*, 2015.
Romans Grecs et Latin, Gallimard, 1958.
Ross, Charles, *Richard III*, 1981.
Rouse, W.H.D., Homer's *The Iliad*, 1938.
Royle, Trevor, *Fighting Mac, The Downfall of Sir Hector Macdonald*.
Ruggiero, Guido, *The Boundaries of Eros*, 1985.
Russo, William/Jan Merlin, *MGM Makes Boys Town*, 2012.

Sabatini Rafael, *The Life of Cesare Borgia*, 1920.

Saint Bris, Gonzague, *Henri IV*, 2009.

Saslow James, *Ganymede in the Renaissance*, 1986.

Sawyer-Lauçanno, *An Invisible Specter, Paul Bowles*, 1989.

Schama, Simon, *Citizens* 1989.

Schiff, Stacy, *Cleopatra*, 2010.

Schom, Alam, *Napoleon Bonaparte*, 1997.

Scurr, Ruth, *Fatal Purity*, 2007.

Setz, Wolfram, *The Sins of the Cities of the Plain*, 1881.

Seward Desmond, *Caravaggio – A Passionate Life*, 1998.

Seymour, Craig, *All I could Bare*, 2008.

Shakespeare, Nicholas, *Bruce Chatwin*, 1999.

Shapiro, James, *1599*, 2005.

Shaw, Aiden, *Sordid Truths*, 2009.

Shelden, Michael, *Graham Greene, The Man Within*, 1994.

Shilts, Randy, *And the Band Played on*, 1987.

Simonetta Marcello, *The Montefeltro Conspiracy*, 2008. Wonderful.

Skidmore, Chris, *Bosworth*, 1988.

Skidmore, *Death and the Virgin*, 2007.

Soares, André, *The Life of Ramon Novarro*, 2010.

Solnon, Jean-François, *Henry III*, 1996.

Spoto, Donald, *The Life of Tennessee Williams,* 1985.

Stewart, Alan, *The Cradle King, A Life of James VI & I*, 2003.

Stirling, Stuart, *Pizarro Conqueror of the Inca*, 2005.

Strathern, Paul, *The Medici, Godfathers of the Renaissance*, 2003.

Strauss Barry, *The Spartacus War*, 2009.

Stuart, Stirling, *Pizarro - Conqueror of the Inca*, 2005.

Suetonius, *The Twelve Caesar.s*

Tacitus, *The Annals of Imperial Rome.*

Tacitus, *The Histories*

Tamagne, Florence, *A History of Homosexuality in Europe*, 2004.

Teeman, Tim, *In Bed with Gore Vidal*, 2013.

Terry, Paul, *In Search of Captain Moonlite*, 2013.

That Man: Peter Berlin, DVD.

Thucydides, *The Peloponnesian War,* Penguin Classics.

Tibullus, *The Elegies of Tibullus*, translated by Theodore C. Williams

Tuchman, Barbara, *A Distant Mirror*, 1978.

Turner, Ralph, *Eleanor of Aquitaine*, 2009.

Unger Miles, *Machiavelli*, 2008.

Unger Miles, *Magnifico, The Brilliant Life and Violent Time.s*

Unger, Harlow Giles, *Lafayette*, 2002.

Unger, Miles, *Machiavelli*, 2008.

Vanderbilt, Arthur, *Best-Kept Boy in the World*, 2014.

Vasari, We would know next to nothing if it were not for him.

Vaughan, Richard, *John the Fearless*, 1973.

Vidal, Gore, *Palimpsest: A Memoir*, 1995.

Virgil, *The Aeneid*, Everyman's Library, Knopf, 1907.

Viroli, Maurizio, *Niccolo's Smile, A Biography of Machiavelli*, 1998.

Walsh, Kenneth M., *wasn't tomorrow wonderful?* 2014.

Ward-Perkins Bryan, *The Fall of Rome*, 2005

Warren, W.L., *Henry II*, 1973.

Watson, Steven, *Factory Made*, 2003.

Weir Alison, The Princes in the Tower, 1992. Marvelous.

Weir, Alison, *Eleanor of Aquitaine*, 1999. Weir is a fabulous writer.

Weir, Alison, *Mary, Queen of Scots*, 2003.

Weir, Alison, *The Princes in the Tower*, 1992. Marvelous.

Weir, Alison, *The Wars of the Roses*, 1995.

Wheaton James, *Spartacus*, 2011.

Whyte, Kenneth, *The Uncrowned King*, 2008.

Wikipedia: Research today is impossible without the aid of this monument.

Williams Craig A. *Roman Homosexuality*, 2010

Williams John, *Augustus*, 1972.

Wilson, Derek, *The Uncrowned Kings of England*, 2005.

Winecoff, Charles, *Anthony Perkins, split image*, 1996.

Wolff, Geoffrey, *Black Sun: The Violent Eclipse of Harry Crosby*, 1976.

Woods, Gregory, *Homintern*, 2016.

Worthington, Ian, *Philip II of Macedonia*, 2008.

Wright Ed, *History's Greatest Scandals*, 2006.

Wroe Ann, *Perking, A Story of Deception*, 2003. Fabulous

Xenophon, *A History of My Time*s, Penguin Classics.

Xenophon, *The Persian Expedition*, 1949.

Zachks, Richard, *History Laid Bare*, 1994.

Zeeland, Steven, *Barrack Buddies and Soldier Lovers*, 1993.

Zeeland, Steven, *Military Trade*, 1999.

Zeeland, Steven, *Sailors and Sexual Identity*, 1995.

Zeeland, Steven, *The Masculine M*arine, 1996.

INDEX